Paleo
Indulgences

Healthy Gluten-Free Recipes to Satisfy Your Primal Cravings

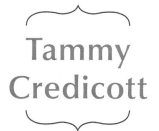

Tammy Credicott

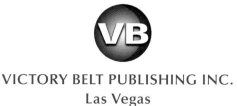

VICTORY BELT PUBLISHING INC.
Las Vegas

Photographs by Tammy Credicott

First Published in 2012 by Victory Belt Publishing

ISBN 13: 978-1-936608-68-3

Printed in the USA

RRD 02-13

Foreword
By Robb Wolf

New York Times bestselling author of *The Paleo Solution*

You might not expect a book describing delectable indulgences to have a foreword detailing life and death. Well, this one does. Almost fifteen years ago I was a mess. I had ulcerative colitis, high blood pressure, depression, and some kind of wacky full-body pain and fatigue that made getting out of bed in the morning seem nearly impossible. I was a ripe, old mid-twenty-something eating what I thought was the bee's knees nutritionally—a high-carb, low-fat, vegan diet full of grains and legumes. Unbeknown to me, I was one of the many, many people for whom these foods are anything but healthy. Through some detective work I figured out that I had a gluten intolerance (celiac disease), as well as sensitivity to almost everything in the grain-legume category. This led to my discovery of the Paleo diet, which completely healed me. It also fired up my passion as a research biochemist and strength-and-conditioning coach to fully explore the benefits and possibilities that Paleo nutrition might have to offer. And that work inspired me to establish a gym (NorCal Strength and Conditioning) that was picked as one of *Men's Health's* thirty best gyms in America, to produce a podcast that is in the top five in the iTunes health category, and to write what became a *New York Times* best-selling book, *The Paleo Solution*.

I think it's safe to say that there is something to the Paleo concept! Even so, although I am grateful for the discoveries that have allowed me to regain my health, for many years my only "treat" was a piece of fruit or perhaps some dark chocolate. Not bad when you consider how sick I was, but sometimes a caveman just wants a little something more. Enter *Paleo Indulgences*. Tammy Credicott has taken her experience as a mom, foodie extraordinaire, and recipe developer for *Paleo Magazine*, and produced a book that could pridefully rest on *any* discerning cook's bookshelf, all while remaining true to the Paleo concepts of grain-, legume-, and (mostly) dairy-free living. The recipes herein run the gamut from simple and tasty to dinner-party-worthy creations. They are all delicious. Tammy introduces you to the basics of Paleo eating, the preferred and less-preferred foods, and then lets loose an extravaganza of good eats. This book is a must-have for anyone living a Paleo or gluten-free lifestyle—plus it's a great way to introduce Paleo/gluten-free treats to folks who might think dessert is not possible if it doesn't involve processed sugar and flour and other unwholesome ingredients.

Enjoy your *Paleo Indulgences!*

Robb Wolf

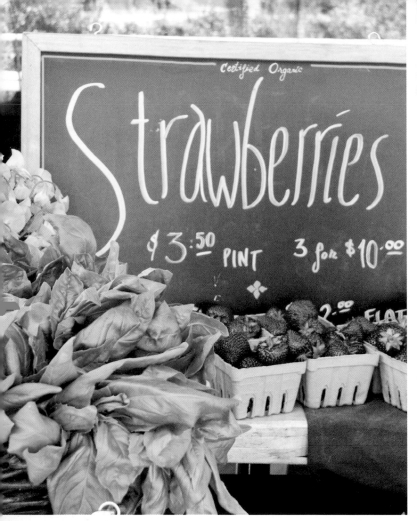

Certified Organic

Strawberries

$3.50 PINT   3 for $10.00

2.00 FLAT

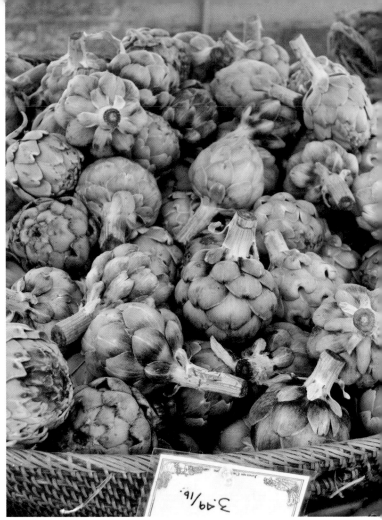

3.49/lb.

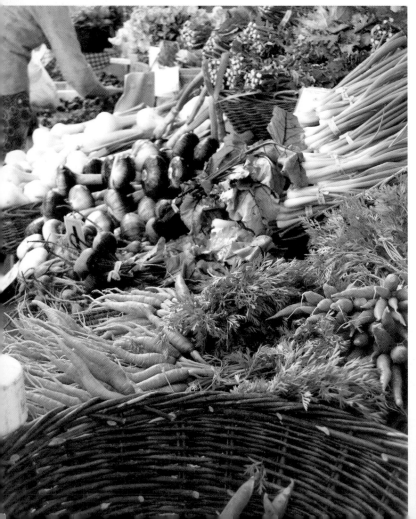

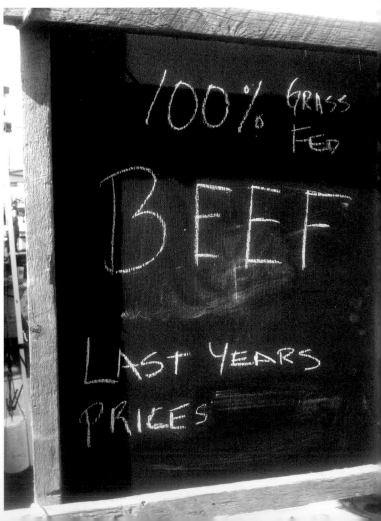

100% GRASS FED

BEEF

LAST YEARS PRICES

Contents

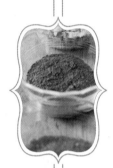

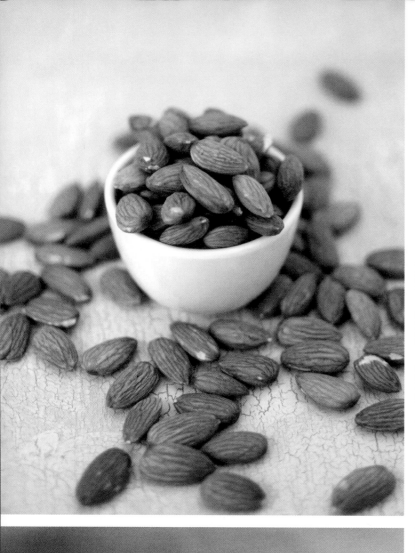
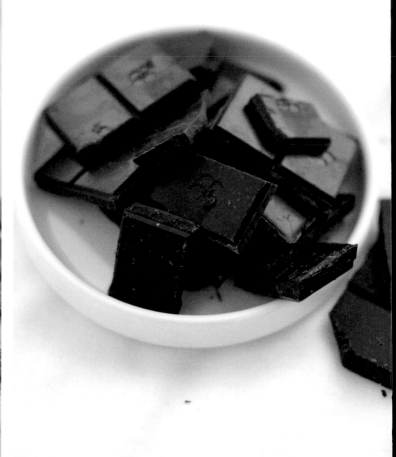
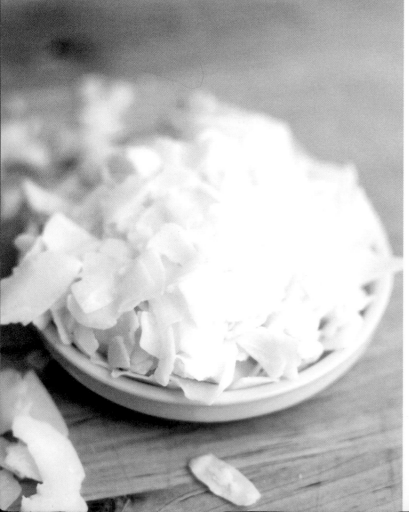
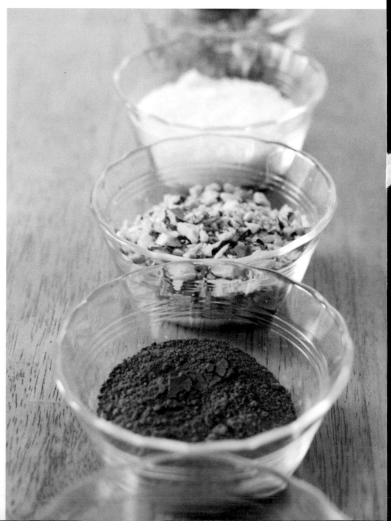

The Bakery

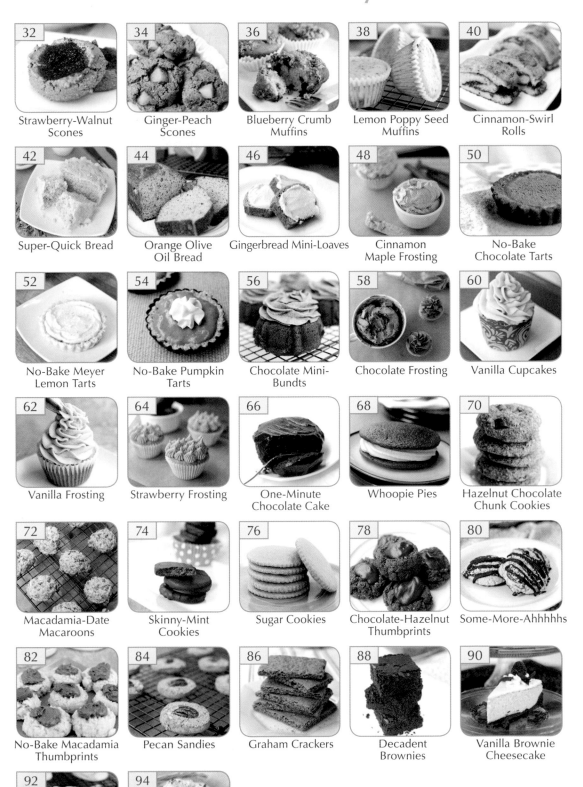

Thumbnail Recipe Table of Contents

Today's Specials

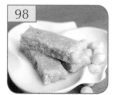
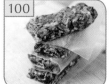
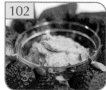
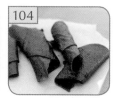
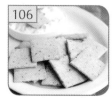
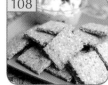
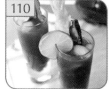
Restaurant Recreations

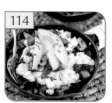
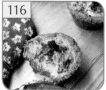
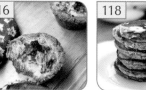
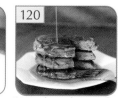
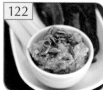
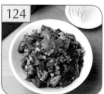
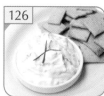
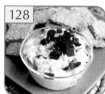
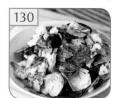
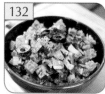
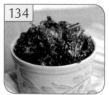
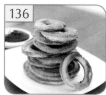
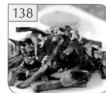
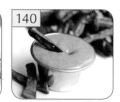
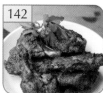
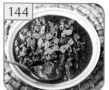
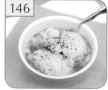
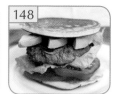
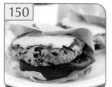
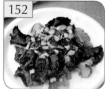

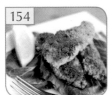
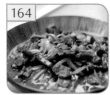
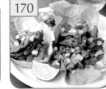
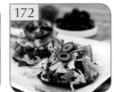
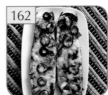
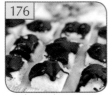
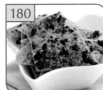
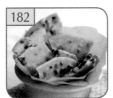
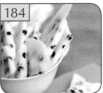
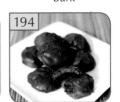
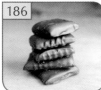
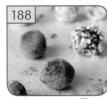
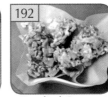

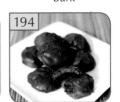
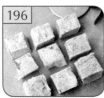
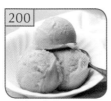
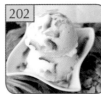
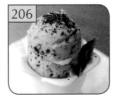
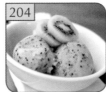
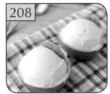
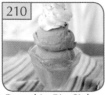
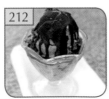
Thumbnail Recipe Table of Contents

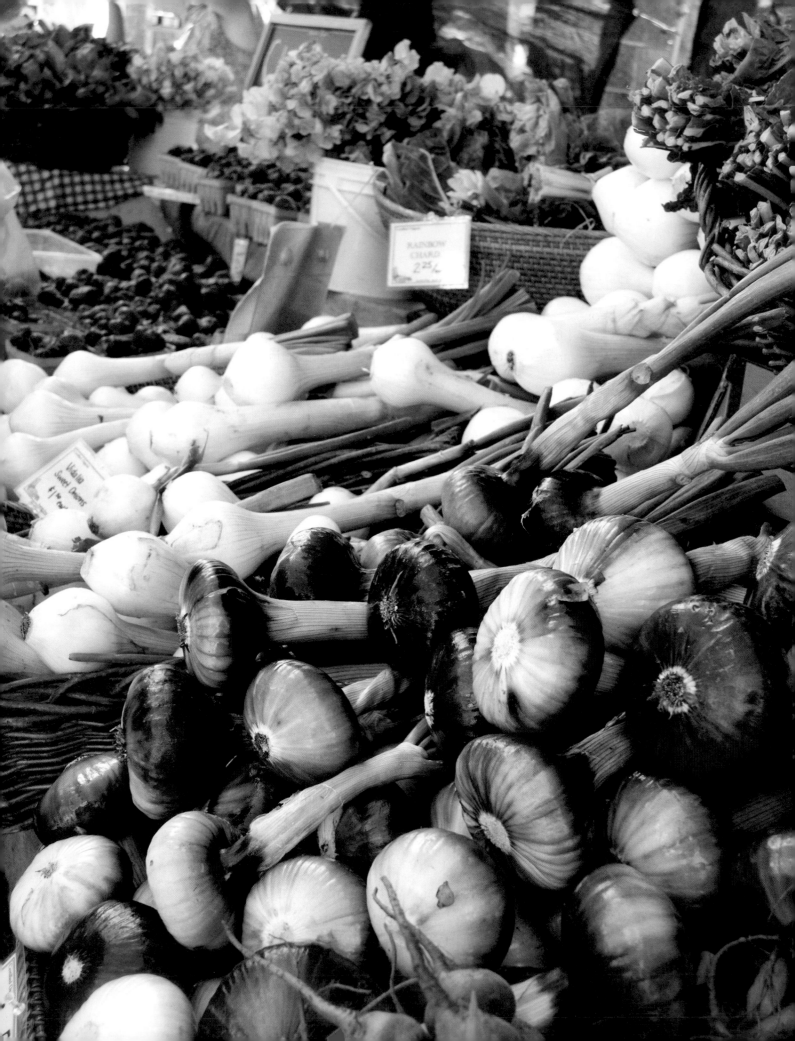

Acknowledgments

Thank you to my amazingly supportive husband for inspiring me every day to be a healthier, better version of myself. A big hug and squeeze to my two amazing daughters for always giving me their honest opinion of my kitchen creations, and for loving me unconditionally each and every day, even when I make something terrible.

A gigantic thank you to Victory Belt Publishing, and especially Erich Krauss, for their support, expertise, and overall coolness. I appreciate the opportunity you've given me to create and eat wonderful food as part of the best job ever!

And thank you to my family, friends, and supporters for showering me with more love and encouragement than I could ever have imagined. I feel lucky and blessed to have each and every one of you in my life!

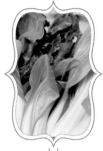

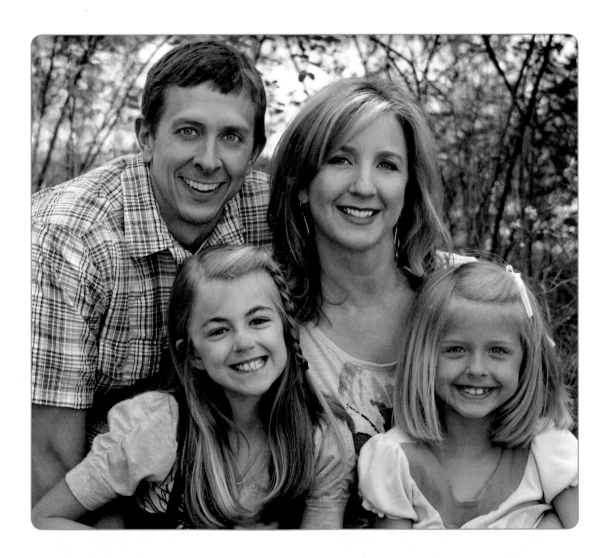

Introduction

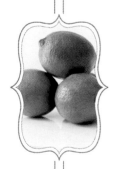

What seems like a million years ago, my husband was diagnosed with celiac disease, as well as dairy, egg, and various other food intolerances. With the research frenzy that followed, we were able to answer many lingering questions about issues our children had been facing, like ADD, eczema, night terrors, and delayed verbal development. The light bulbs had been switched on. Our family had food allergies.

Prior to this revelation, my husband and I had always tried to take a healthier path in our life together. We worked out religiously. We ate lots of lean meat, mostly in the form of boneless, skinless chicken breasts, veggies, as little fat as possible, and lots of fruits and whole grains. Healthy, right? Unfortunately, this diet led to the explosion of problems my family was experiencing. The very same grains and ultra-low fat foods that were being touted as "healthy" were making us all sick. We were just lucky enough to have bodies that told us this was wrong before our health deteriorated further. Millions of others are unknowingly facing heart disease, cancers, and autoimmune diseases because they don't realize that there is a vital link between what they eat and their health.

After my husband's celiac diagnosis we changed our family's diet to gluten-free, dairy-free, and egg-free, so that we could all eat together without the additional work and anxiety that came with preparing separate meals. This led us, eventually, to dip our toes into the ever-popular vegan-diet pool. Again, the media and experts were raving about its benefits, and we needed to get healthy, so it seemed to make sense. This experiment lasted about six months, because at the end of this period the kids were worse than ever, my husband was still sick, and I had gained ten pounds and was so tired I could hardly make it through the day without a nap. This was not the miracle we had been looking for. Thankfully, in my husband's quest to find answers, he found the Paleo diet.

Almost immediately he started to gain healthy weight. He wasn't in the bathroom constantly, and normal color returned to his previously gray face. I was getting my husband back! I decided I needed to give this diet a try and be supportive of his efforts, so I read about and studied the Paleo/primal lifestyle and jumped in with both feet.

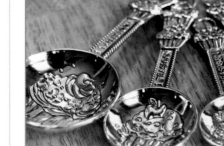

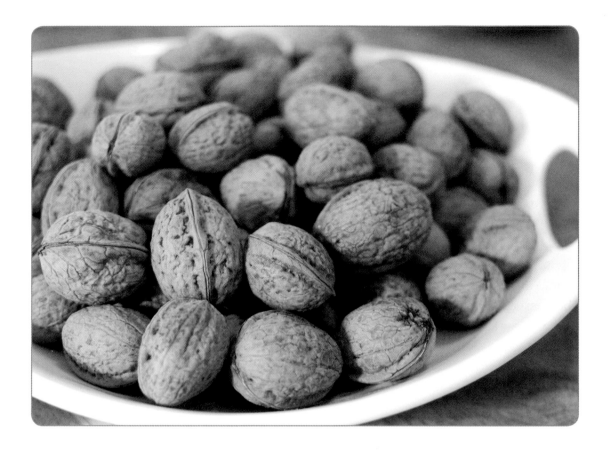

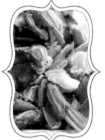

My first week was rocky, to say the least. Even though I'd been gluten-free for quite a while, I now realized how heavily I'd relied on gluten-free grains and sugar as the bulk of my daily diet. That first week my body was literally aching for more grains—a quick fix for my plummeting blood sugar. But after a week or so, I lost about five pounds, my skin was clear, and I regained mental clarity I'd forgotten was possible. No more brain fog. Wow! I haven't looked back since, and I honestly haven't felt this good in probably twenty years. I lost twenty-seven pounds in about seven months and went down three clothing sizes. Plus, I sleep soundly and wake up refreshed, something that eluded me in the past decade.

My journey is still in progress, though, and I'm not sure where my weight or clothing size will level off. But every day I learn something new about this way of living. Our Paleo lifestyle is definitely one that changes and grows with the knowledge we gain from the new information constantly available to us. We believe that every individual is different and that you must listen to your body and know what works for you. Even foods within the Paleo realm can be bothersome for some folks and fine for others. For example, nuts and full-fat coconut milk cause some intestinal distress for my husband and youngest daughter. My oldest daughter and I seem to tolerate them just fine, in moderation. So remember to listen to your body and make adjustments as you go, especially if you have food allergies and intolerances. Paleo in and of itself is not a "one size fits all" way of eating. Which brings me to why I wrote *Paleo Indulgences*.

About the Book

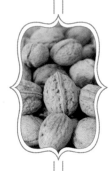

The intention of *Paleo Indulgences* is not to say, "Hey, look at all the crap you can get away with eating on a Paleo diet!" The aim is to present options for better choices when you just have to have that special treat. Let's face it: Life happens, cravings happen, special occasions happen. You don't have to feel guilty about going a bit off-plan; just make the best choice possible and move on. You don't have to eat the "real deal," which will put you back at square one with sugar cravings, carb cravings, and inflammation. You don't have to undo all you've worked so hard for! There is an alternative.

It goes without saying, but I will say it anyway, *Paleo Indulgences* is not a daily guide on how to eat a primal diet. By no means am I going to tell you to devour sweets and treats every day. *Paleo Indulgences* is a tool to help you stay on track by providing better choices for occasional treats that are still Paleo-friendly. My husband and I have heard many people in the Paleo community talk about their occasional "cheats," like pizza, doughnuts, hamburgers (with bun), and cookies. Not healthy versions mind you, but the typical sugar-loaded, gluten-filled ones. On the flip side, we also talk to many people in the Paleo community who are so strict that they never touch a drop of any kind of sweetener, nor do they allow their kids to indulge in anything that contains carbs. For my family, I felt we needed a middle ground.

I believe you can be Paleo and have a brownie once in a blue moon. I believe you can live a primal lifestyle and still bake cookies with your kids at Christmas. I also believe that you should make these brownies and cookies using the highest-quality Paleo-acceptable ingredients and that they should look and taste amazing. I'm not an advocate of cheating at any point with gluten. Ever. It causes inflammation, which takes a long time to get out of your system. Plus, for most people, it causes feelings and cravings from the past to resurface with a vengeance. Why do that to yourself over and over again? Partake in the occasional sweet treat or fried goody, but do it only occasionally, and make it a Paleo version.

Another reason for writing *Paleo Indulgences* was to hopefully show those who say Paleo is difficult and super-restrictive that they are wrong. Quite the contrary, this is by far the easiest way of eating I've ever encountered. No more shopping for hours, scouring the entire grocery store for "healthy" foods. What's easier than buying beautiful grass-fed meat and fresh, organic veggies? I'm in and out of the store in no time! I also wanted to share with people how delicious, nutritious, and special the food can be. I wanted to show them that they won't be ostracized for not indulging at the next social gathering—not when they show up with a cupcake that looks like the real thing but isn't full of gluten and sugar and who knows what else.

For those still shaking their heads because they think that any self-respecting Paleo person would never eat a treat, I say, *what works for you may not work for everyone else.* Everyone's life is different, and we should all strive to be more understanding of that. My philosophy is that it's one thing to model our diet after our ancestors, but it's not feasible to try to recreate the entire caveman lifestyle. I like my food processor, toilet, and bed way too much. The fact is, we live in a modern society; we encounter modern struggles, stresses, and conveniences; and our environment and food sources are nowhere near the same as they were 100 years ago, let alone 10,000 years ago. We live social lives and celebrate birthdays, holidays, and anniversaries. We attend barbecues, potlucks, and school functions. Socializing is as important to our overall well-being as the food we eat and how much sleep we get. And socializing inevitably involves food. This book is designed to help you enjoy gathering with friends and family while still staying on track nutritionally—and show the world that living a Paleo lifestyle doesn't mean you have to sit in the corner at the next family reunion with nothing but a chicken leg!

I've come to realize that the people who stick with dietary changes generally baby-step it toward better nutrition rather than dive-bomb into it. I wanted

Paleo Indulgences to be a tool to help those trying to make better food choices by providing recipes for tasty Paleo alternatives to familiar comfort foods. Because, shockingly, I have yet to convert anyone to a Paleo lifestyle by screaming about what he or she can NEVER eat again. I wanted to show that there is a middle ground; that you don't have to turn your back on life as you have known it; that you don't have to be perfect every second of the day; that you can still put dessert on your holiday table and make cupcakes for your child's birthday.

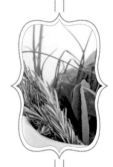

I have organized the book around some of the most common pitfalls for a Paleo lifestyle. In this way, you will find help to stay strong in places that would just love to sabotage your resolve, such as: "The Bakery," "The Candy Counter," and "The Ice Cream Shop." I will also arm you with lots of "Restaurant Recreations" and "Today's Specials," so you won't be tempted to go off the deep end with the standard fare. *Paleo Indulgences* will get you through the 20 percent of your life when you're craving a dish from your past or you're celebrating a special occasion, without taking a bite out of the hard work you put in the other 80 percent of the time. Be mindful of what you eat, enjoy each and every bite, and then, go ahead and indulge every so often. Just do it responsibly, with *Paleo Indulgences!*

What Is Paleo/Primal?

Call it Paleo or primal—the essence is the same. It means nourishing our bodies with foods we were evolutionarily designed to eat. This means primarily foods that were consumed by our hunter-gatherer ancestors prior to the agricultural revolution. Among the foods they did not typically consume were grains, sugar, legumes, and processed foods. Grains have been scientifically proven to be gut irritants, especially those containing gluten: they are highly inflammatory, and inflammation also causes a host of other modern health problems, such as diabetes and heart disease.

There is a wealth of information available on the science behind the Paleo/primal lifestyle, and I encourage you to read as much as you can. Understanding what our modern, processed foods do to your body will change your outlook on what society deems "healthy" (which hasn't worked so far so why do we keep listening to it?) and will change your life for the better. Here are some great places to start:

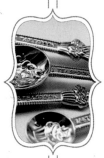

Get to Know Paleo

Robb Wolf – Check out his New York Times bestselling book, *The Paleo Solution* and learn the "why's" of the Paleo lifestyle. He presents the science of the diet with a sense of humor and in terms that are easy to understand and apply. www.robbwolf.com

Mark Sisson – Mark's book, *The Primal Blueprint*, will give you the step by step guide you need when you ask yourself, "What do I do first?" His laid back style for life is contagious and will give you a whole new appreciation for learning to be a kid again. www.marksdailyapple.com

Nora Gedgaudas – Author of *Primal Body, Primal Mind*, she goes in depth as to what those processed carbs are really doing inside your body, and more importantly your brain. www.primalbody-primalmind.com

Paleo Magazine - *Paleo Magazine* is the first, and only, magazine dedicated to the Paleo lifestyle and ancestral health. This bi-monthly print publication is packed with the latest research, exercise and nutrition. Also included are interviews, inspirational stories, recipes, reviews, info on raising Paleo kids and much more. www.paleomagonline.com

Cookbooks, Blogs & Websites – Oh my! –There is an amazing amount of information out there on how to live your best Paleo life...way too many to list here. Just Google "Paleo" and spend some time getting acquainted with some of these wonderful resources.

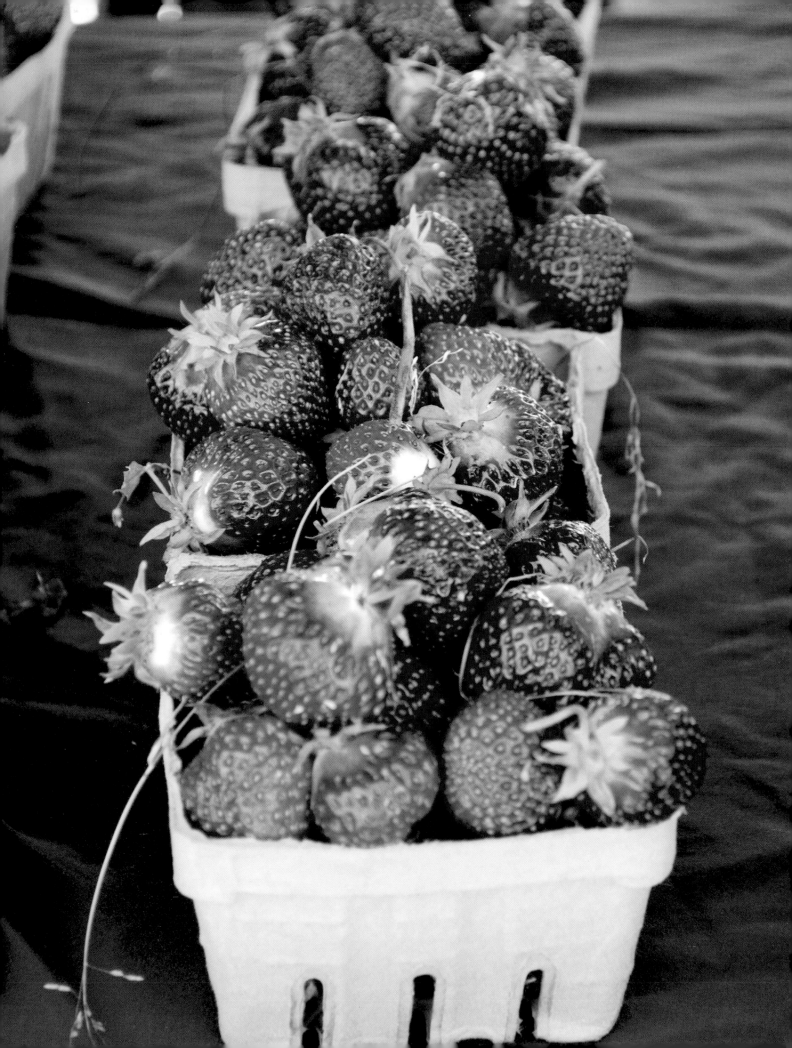

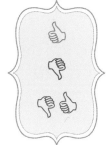

The Do's and Don'ts

Do's

Fish/Seafood

Healthy, Natural Fats

Nuts, Seeds

Organic Fruits

Organic Veggies

Pastured/Grass-Fed Meats

Don'ts

Grains

Legumes

Processed Foods

Soy

Refined Sugar

Gray Areas

Alcohol – Every once in a while, a glass is o.k. But no regular beer, which contains gluten.

Condiments – To make or to buy, that is the question! My family doesn't use ketchup, mayo, or Worcestershire sauce enough to merit making our own. We'd create too much waste by throwing away unused portions of the necessary ingredients. For us, it makes sense to purchase the highest-quality condiments we can find. Look for organic versions with no soy or sugar added, when possible. If I can't find a sugar-free version for, say, Worcestershire sauce, I don't freak out, because the little I use here and there isn't going to derail my Paleo progress. If you want to be really strict and make your own ketchup and mayo, check out the websites I've noted throughout the book which have some fantastic recipes.

Dairy – For anyone with autoimmune issues, or those trying to lose weight, dairy should be eliminated or reduced. If you choose to consume dairy, choose organic full-fat products from pastured cows to maximize nutrients. There's lots of talk in the Paleo community about raw dairy. I recommend doing your research on the benefits and risks of raw dairy and making your own, informed decision about whether it's right for you and your family.

Natural Sweeteners – Used in moderation, natural sweeteners can satisfy sweet cravings and potentially provide some health benefits. Choose organic, raw, local honey; pure, organic maple syrup; or coconut crystals/nectar (a.k.a. palm sugar). However, if you're looking to lean out, you will want to skip the sweets for a while.

The 80/20 Philosophy

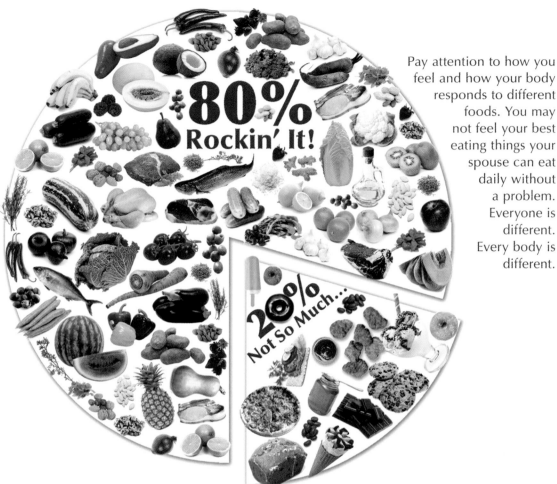

Pay attention to how you feel and how your body responds to different foods. You may not feel your best eating things your spouse can eat daily without a problem. Everyone is different. Every body is different.

The 80/20 rule in Paleo means that if you work hard and eat right 80 percent of the time, then the other 20 percent of the time you should be able to cut yourself some slack. This doesn't mean you should gorge on gluten-filled, preservative-laden frozen pizza for this 20%; it just means that you don't have to stress about being perfect every single second of your life.

Another thing to keep in mind regarding this rule is your own individual goals and body type. My husband, who has celiac disease and other food intolerances, is intent on healing his gut and overall health, so he's pretty strict 99 percent of the time. He doesn't have the luxury of being less stringent more often because he doesn't feel well if he eats non-Paleo. Now, my kids live the 80/20 life. They attend school functions, birthday parties, and play dates, so they tend to have Paleo-friendly treats more often. Their young, active bodies can more than handle this higher carb level, so we don't worry about healthy treats, as long as they aren't a daily occurrence. As for me? Well, my body loves carbs and sweets, so when I indulge I generally hold on to every last calorie. I have to be more of a 90/10 eater because otherwise I don't feel my best, and I gain weight.

Ingredients

Here are some of the main ingredients used in *Paleo Indulgences*. This is by no means an all-inclusive list, but it will give you an idea of the main players in the recipes to help you with your shopping. Please refer to individual recipes for specific ingredients.

Protein

Grass-fed, pastured animals are eating a diet they were designed to eat, which means higher quality, better flavor, and more nutrients for us. Check out the resource section in the back of the book for help tracking down pastured, organic meat in your area, including:

- Beef
- Chicken
- Eggs
- Fish, wild-caught, mild white fish (like cod or halibut)
- Pork, including nitrate- or nitrite- and sugar-free bacon

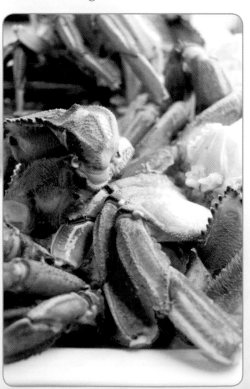

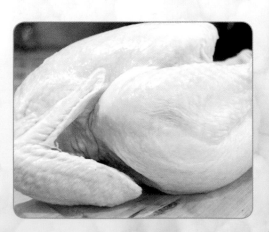

Fats

Because of its health benefits and the decadent and satisfying nature of coconut oil, I use it for most of my cooking and baking. I use more-refined coconut oil for savory cooking because it has a neutral flavor and a higher cooking temperature. I keep raw coconut oil on hand for its higher lauric acid profile and its slightly coconutty flavor, which enhances many desserts and veggies. Plus, it makes a great moisturizer and smells amazing!

Coconut oils are all made from the meat (white flesh) of a mature coconut. Water, fiber, and proteins are removed from the flesh to obtain the oil. Coconut oil is more stable than any other oil because it is predominantly composed of medium-chain fatty acids (MCFAs), which are "saturated" by hydrogen atoms and resist oxidation and, therefore, rancidity. Coconut oil is easily digestible and is sent directly to the liver, where it's converted into energy rather than being stored as fat. It can help stimulate the body's metabolism and is very high in lauric acid (the predominant type of MCFA in coconut oil), which can help strengthen the immune system.

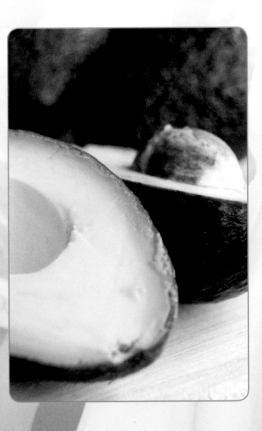

- Avocados
- Coconut butter
- Coconut milk (canned, full-fat or light)
- Coconut oil
- Cream cheese
- Extra-virgin olive oil
- Mascarpone cheese
- Olives
- Palm shortening
- Sour cream
- Unsweetened coconut flakes and shredded coconut

Ingredients

Veggies and Fruits (a.k.a. Carbs)

Always choose local, organic and in season produce when possible. Of course, there are many more fruits and veggies available that you should partake in. These are just the ones I used frequently in *Paleo Indulgences*.

- Bananas
- Broccoli
- Carrots
- Celery
- Cucumbers
- Dates

- Garlic
- Green onions
- Greens (kale, lettuces)
- Kiwi
- Onions

- Oranges
- Raisins
- Strawberries
- Sweet potatoes
- Tomatoes
- Zucchini

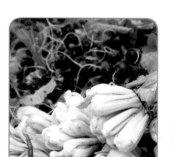
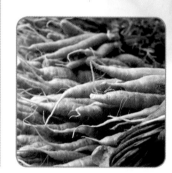
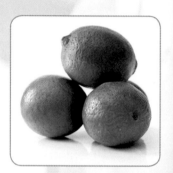

Nuts and Seeds

I list nuts and seeds separately from fats because, although they should be in the fat category, they should not be your main source of fat. Nuts and seeds tend to be higher in omega-6s, and we are striving for higher levels of omega-3s to get more in-line with our historical intake of a 1:1, omega-6 to omega-3 ratio. This is why I consider them a snack, an extra—not a primary source of fat or protein.

- Almonds (including almond butter)
- Cashews
- Hazelnuts

- Macadamia nuts
- Pumpkin seeds
- Sunflower seeds
- Walnuts

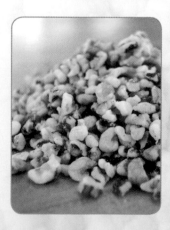

Natural Sweeteners

· Pure Maple Syrup

Maple syrup is a fairly benign sweetener with potential health benefits, and it is very low in fructose (only about 2 percent). Maple syrup contains less sugar, 17 times more calcium, 11 times more magnesium, 6½ times more zinc, and 4 times more potassium than honey. However, it should be noted that the sugar and mineral content in maple syrup can vary depending on the tree it is taken from and where and when the syrup is produced.

I often use pure maple syrup in my baking for its great flavor and high level of sweetness, which means I can use less and still achieve the taste I'm looking for. I also like it because since sap is subjected to heat to create syrup, maple syrup doesn't deteriorate during the baking process.

· Organic Honey

Honey has been shown to possess antibacterial and antimicrobial

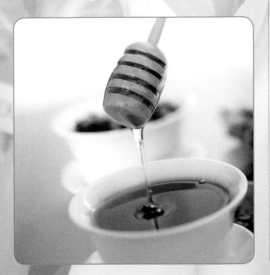

properties, and it may help protect against cardiovascular disease as well. Honey has also been shown to lower triglycerides and fasting blood sugar levels. And while it has a high fructose level, studies have shown that substituting honey for fructose may protect against the pro-oxidative effects of the fructose. Theoretically, the fructose in honey may be less problematic for those with fructose issues.

Not all honey is created equal, so it is important to shop around. Translucent honey, found in traditional bear containers at your supermarket, doesn't have the same health benefits as raw honey, because of the over-processing. Whenever possible, use raw, organic honey, as it will provide the maximum health benefits. Also, the flavor of honey is dependent on the flower its nectar comes from, and can range from subtle to overwhelming. To my palate, clover honey tends to have a stronger flavor than I prefer, and so I avoid using it in cooking and baking.

· Coconut Nectar

Coconut nectar is a low glycemic sweetener derived from the sap of coconut blossoms. It's chock-full of vitamins, minerals, amino acids, and other nutrients (including vitamin C) and has a low fructose content. Compared with traditional brown sugar, coconut nectar has

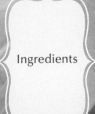

Ingredients

20 times the nitrogen, 26 times the phosphorus, 15 times the potassium, 10 times the zinc, and 1½ times the iron. Coconut nectar is minimally processed at a low temperature to remove excess moisture which allows the sap to thicken.

Taken a step further, when coconut nectar is air-dried, coconut crystals are formed (also known as palm sugar), which can be used like traditional sugar. It is also low-glycemic and nutrient-rich. And since both sweeteners are completely unrefined, unbleached, non-GMO, gluten-free, and still contain key vitamins and minerals, they are both well used in my kitchen.

Grain-Free Flours

- Almond flour
- Arrowroot starch
- Coconut flour

- Hazelnut flour
- Walnut meal
- Tapioca Starch

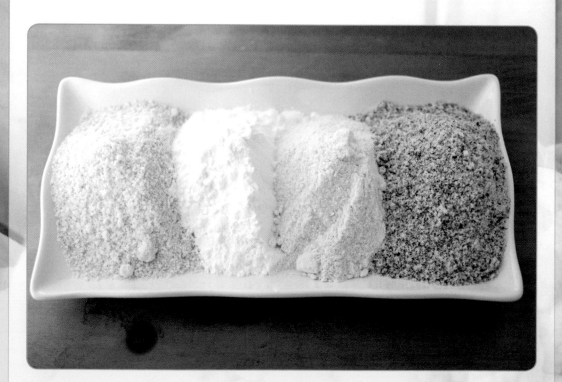

Miscellaneous

- Any and all dried spices

- Canned tomato sauce, tomato paste, diced tomatoes (organic and non-BPA cans)

- Chicken and beef stock, preferably homemade

- Coconut aminos

- Dark chocolate (72 percent or darker), preferably without added soy or dairy

- Fish sauce

- Fresh herbs (dill, chives, sage, rosemary)

- Freshly ground black pepper

- Gelatin

- Raw apple cider vinegar

- Sea salt

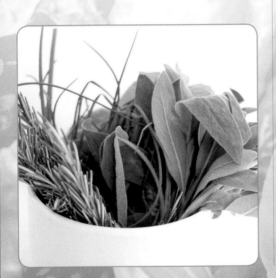
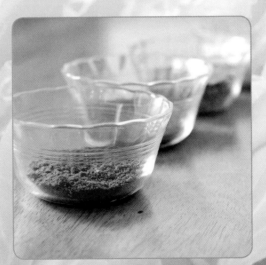

Ingredients

Freedom to Choose

All of the recipes in *Paleo Indulgences* are free of wheat, gluten, grains, peanuts, and soy. To help you choose recipes that work for additional food intolerances or allergies you may have, each is labeled indicating whether it is also free of any of the other most common food allergens.

Dairy Free

Egg Free

Nut Free

Fish Free

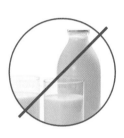

Dairy Free

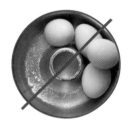

Egg Free

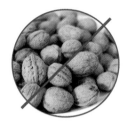

Nut Free
(excluding coconut)

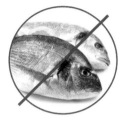

Fish Free/
Shellfish Free

Here's the Deal ...

1. For all ingredients, buy organic, local, fair trade, pastured, grass-fed, and as unprocessed as possible.

2. Almond flour and almond meal are not the same thing. Almond meal is more coarsely ground and generally, but not always, includes the skin of the almond. Almond flour is made from blanched, finely ground nuts. The difference between the two is huge when it comes to baking. Unfortunately, the almond meal/flour from Bob's Red Mill, while more readily available, is not ground finely enough, and so I consider it a meal, not a flour. In a pinch, you can sift Bob's and use only the sifted portion.

3. Measure coconut flour as per the recipe and then sift it into a bowl. Coconut flour MUST be sifted prior to mixing it in the recipe or you will have more lumps than you can handle. Trust me, I almost lost an arm trying to mix out all the lumps the first time I used coconut flour.

4. To cut down on sugar when a recipe calls for melted chocolate, combine a good-quality dark chocolate (I use Trader Joe's 72% dark) with an unsweetened (100% cacao) dark chocolate (Dagoba has a great one). This way, you get that rich chocolaty taste without the excess sugar!

5. Because this book is designed for the occasional indulgence, the recipes do not yield huge quantities. If you're baking for a crowd, you can easily double any of the recipes. Just adjust your pan size, and sometimes your bake time, accordingly: more food in the oven absorbing heat means it'll take a little longer to bake.

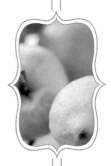

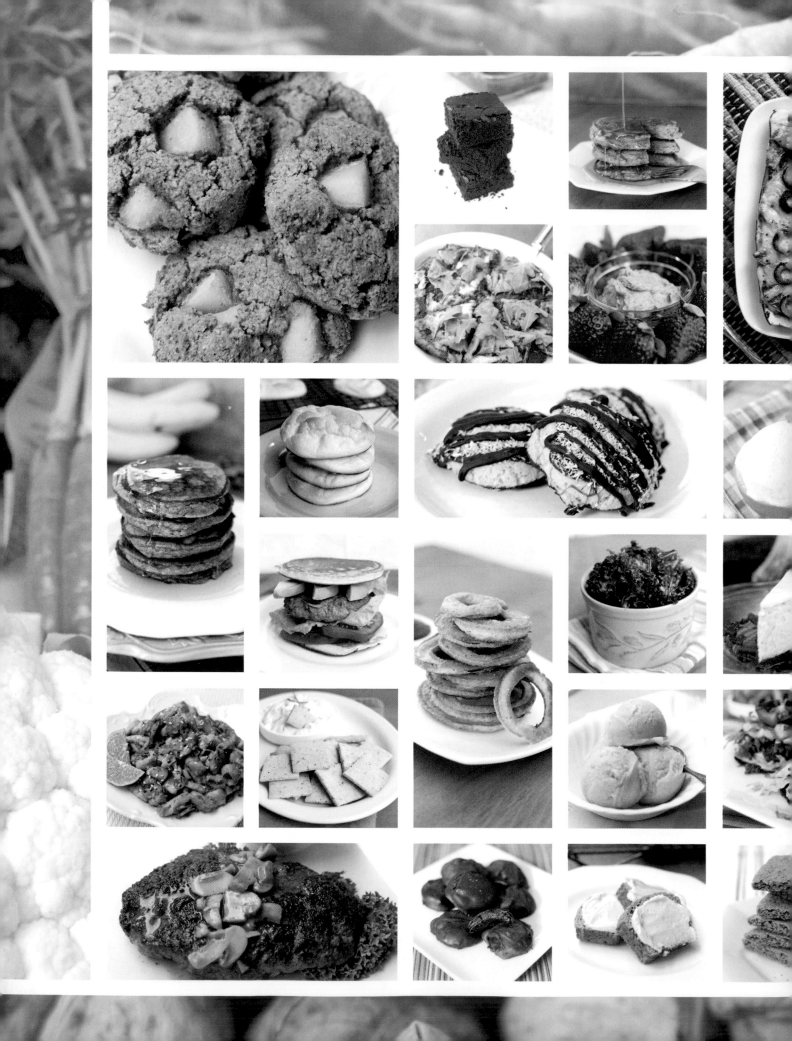

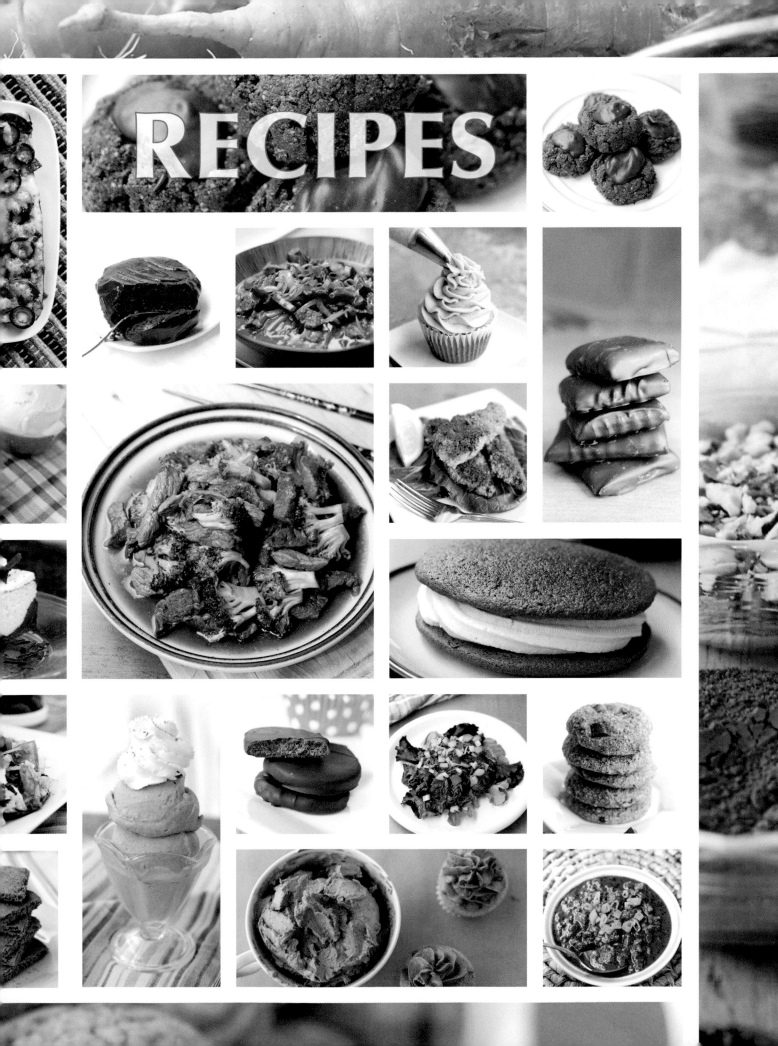

RECIPES

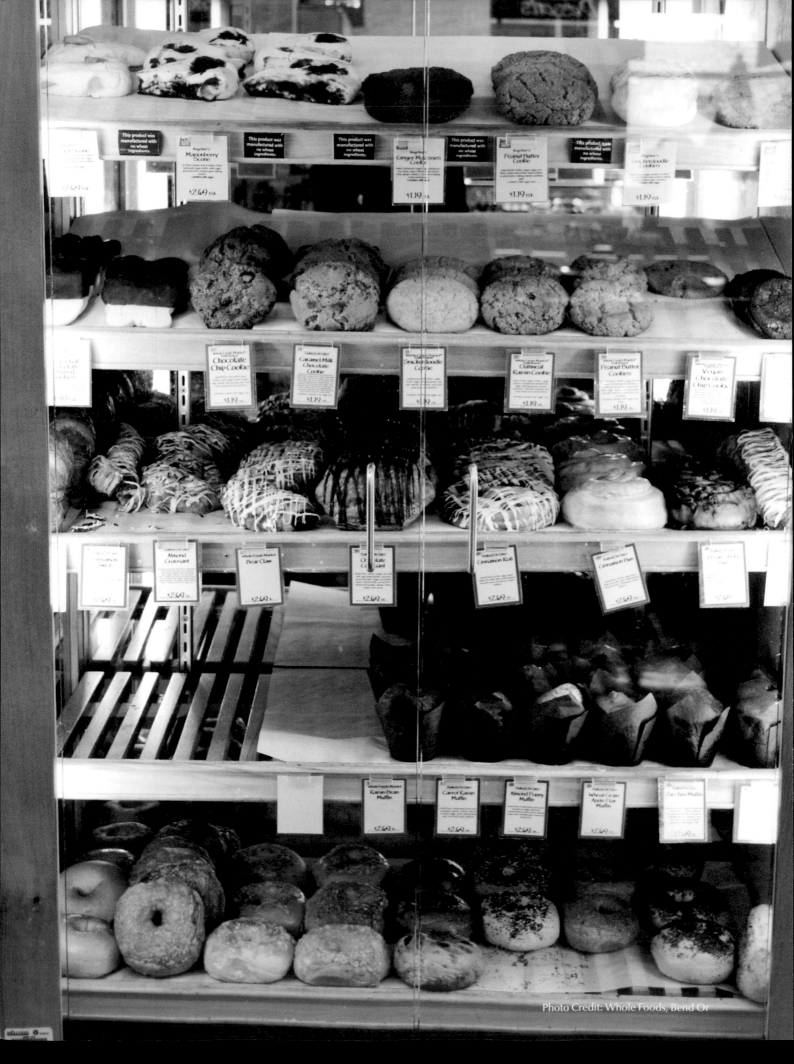

The Bakery

Strawberry-Walnut Scones

Makes 8 scones
Dairy Free • Fish Free

Dry Ingredients

2 cups (300 g) raw walnuts

¼ cup (25 g) coconut flour, sifted

1 tsp cinnamon

1 tsp baking soda

½ tsp sea salt

Wet Ingredients

¼ cup (60 mL) pure maple syrup

1 tsp pure vanilla extract

2 eggs

¼ cup (60 mL) coconut oil, melted

Add On

Sugar-free (100% fruit) strawberry jam

Just right for a special-occasion breakfast or brunch, these tasty scones will win over a crowd. Crispy on the edges, soft and flavorful inside, with a touch of sweet from the jam, they will have you wondering if you just fell off the Paleo wagon! But with no gluten, grains, or cane sugar, you can feel good about this tasty morning treat. Even better—they freeze wonderfully, so they are ready when you are. I like to bring a few in a cooler when we travel, then I just heat and serve with some precooked bacon or sausage for a filling, on-the-go breakfast!

1. Preheat the oven to 350°F.

2. Place the walnuts in a food processor and pulse until a fine meal is formed.

3. Place the walnut meal and the remaining dry ingredients in a medium bowl and whisk to combine.

4. Add the wet ingredients, except the coconut oil, to the walnut meal mixture. Blend well with a hand mixer.

5. With mixer on low, slowly pour in the coconut oil. Mix well.

6. Using an ice-cream size scoop, make 8 even balls of dough and place on a parchment-lined baking sheet. With your thumb, or a teaspoon, make a deep well in the center of each scone.

7. Fill each well with 1 teaspoon strawberry jam.

8. Bake 23-25 minutes, or until tops are golden brown and the dough springs back when pressed lightly.

9. Cool on pans for 5 minutes, then remove to wire racks to cool completely. Store leftovers in an airtight container up to 3 days, or freeze up to 3 months.

Notes:
Try other flavors of your favorite sugar-free jam, such as blackberry or peach!

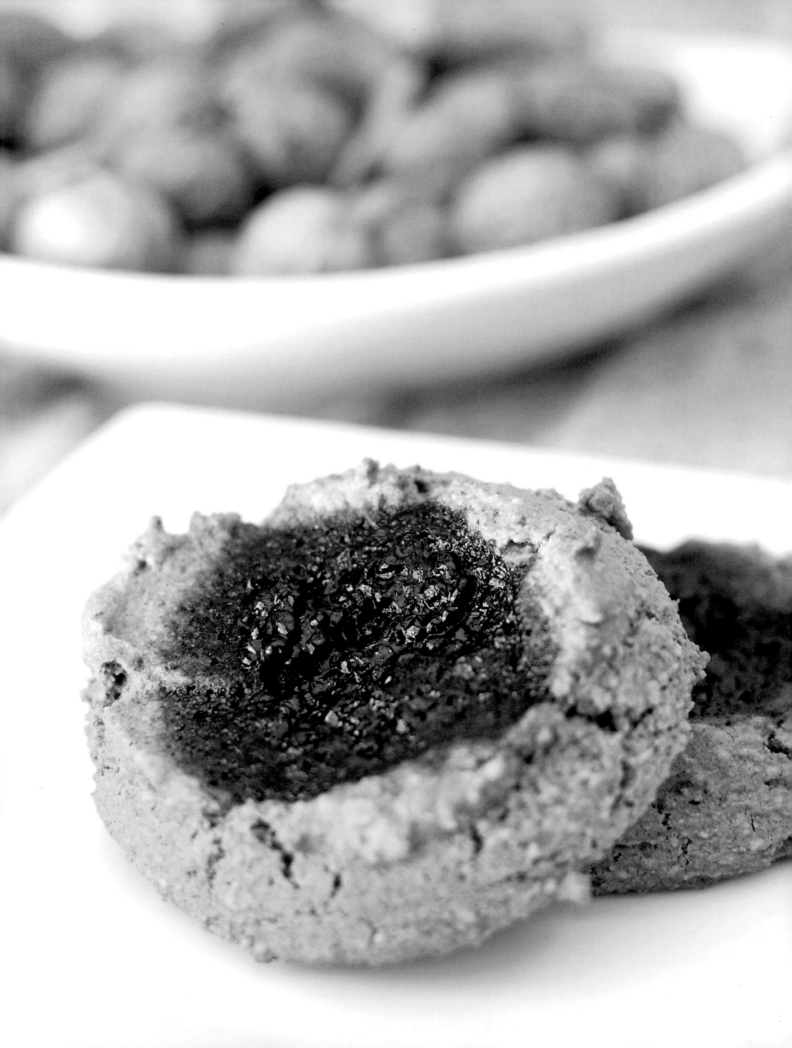

Ginger-Peach Scones

Makes 8 scones
Dairy Free • Fish Free

Dry Ingredients

1½ cups (135 g) almond flour

¼ cup (25 g) coconut flour, sifted

½ tsp cinnamon

1 tsp baking soda

½ tsp sea salt

Wet Ingredients

¼ cup (60 mL) pure maple syrup

1 tsp pure vanilla extract

2 eggs

1½ tsp minced fresh ginger

3 TBSP (45 mL) coconut oil, melted

Add In

1 cup (150 g) coarsely chopped peaches

The fragrant combination of fresh ginger and peaches really makes these scones refreshingly unique. And with such simple, wholesome ingredients, they are easily adapted to fit the tastes of your family! Try adding more or less ginger, or add a cup of chopped pecans to the batter for a little extra crunch. Delicious!

1. Preheat the oven to 350°F.
2. Place the dry ingredients in a medium bowl and whisk to combine.
3. Add the wet ingredients, except the coconut oil, to the dry mixture. Blend well with a hand mixer.
4. With mixer on low, slowly pour in the coconut oil. Mix well.
5. Stir in the peaches.
6. Using an ice-cream size scoop, drop 8 even scoops of dough onto a parchment-lined baking sheet.
7. Bake 23-25 minutes, or until firm and golden brown.
8. Cool on wire racks. Serve! Store leftovers in an airtight container up to 3 days, or freeze up to 3 months.

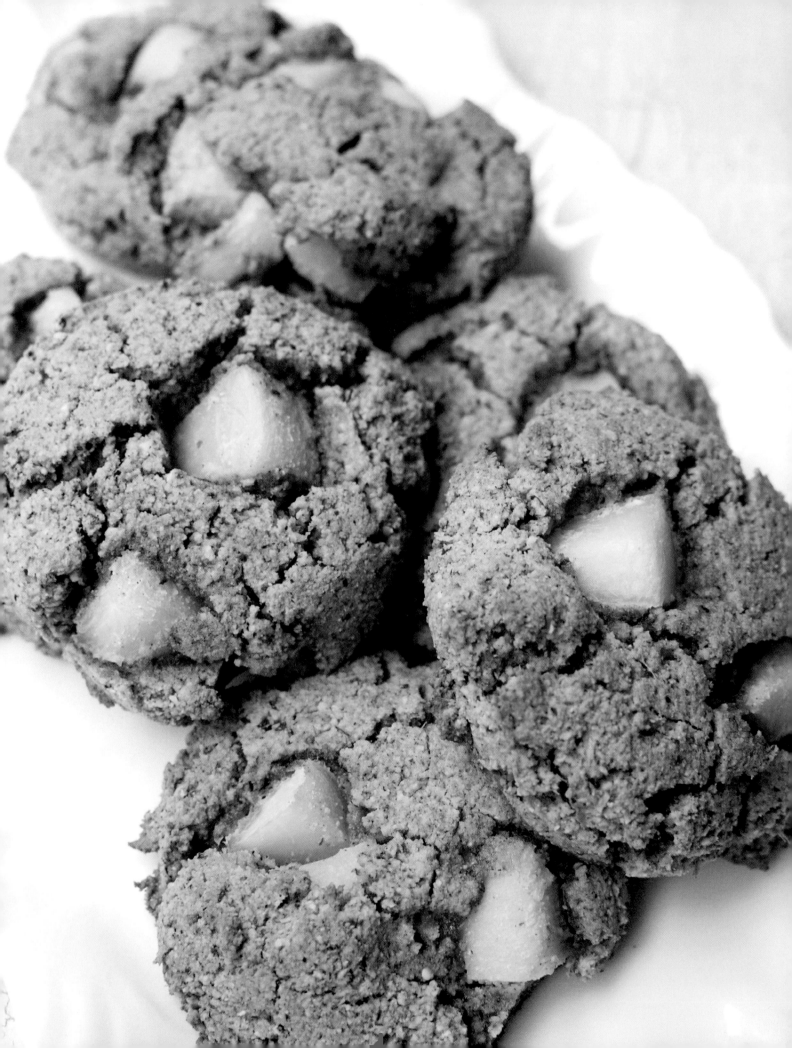

Blueberry Crumb Muffins

Makes 6 muffins

Dairy Free • Nut Free* • Fish Free

Dry Ingredients

⅓ cup (35 g) coconut flour, sifted

¼ tsp sea salt

½ tsp baking powder

⅛ tsp cinnamon

Wet Ingredients

4 eggs

½ tsp pure vanilla extract

¼ cup (60 mL) pure maple syrup

¼ cup (60 mL) coconut milk (full-fat or light)

¼ cup (60 mL) coconut oil, melted

Add In

½ cup (75 g) fresh, wild blueberries (frozen works too, but you'll need to defrost them, and then your batter will be blue—not the prettiest, but still yummy!)

*Optional Crumb Topping

2 TBSP almond meal (Bob's Red Mill is o.k.)

¼ cup (40 g) coarsely chopped raw nuts and seeds (almond, pecan, pumpkin and/or sunflower)

1 TBSP pure maple syrup

1 TBSP coconut oil, melted

Pinch sea salt

I really feel there are a few classic recipes that everyone should have in their kitchen arsenal, and blueberry muffins are definitely at the top of that list! Whether you're simply gluten-free or are now living the Paleo life, a good blueberry muffin can take you through Sunday breakfasts, family brunches, or a Christmas morning if need be. These muffins are soft, fluffy, and bursting with fragrant blueberries. Plus, if you're feeling naughty, the optional crumb topping adds a contrasting crunch. What's not to love?

1. Preheat the oven to 350°F.

2. Place the dry ingredients in a medium bowl and whisk to combine.

3. Add the wet ingredients, except the coconut oil, to the dry and blend well with a hand mixer.

4. With mixer on low, slowly pour in the coconut oil. Blend well.

5. Fold in the blueberries.

6. If desired, make the crumb topping by placing all the topping ingredients in a small bowl and stirring to combine. It should be slightly crumbly.

7. Fill 6 paper-lined muffin cups two-thirds full with batter.

8. Sprinkle 1 teaspoon crumb topping evenly on each muffin.

9. Bake about 30 minutes, or until the center of each muffin springs back to the touch or a toothpick inserted in the center comes out clean. The tops should be golden brown.

10. Cool 5-10 minutes in the pan. Serve! Store any leftovers in an airtight container up to 3 days, or freeze up to 3 months.

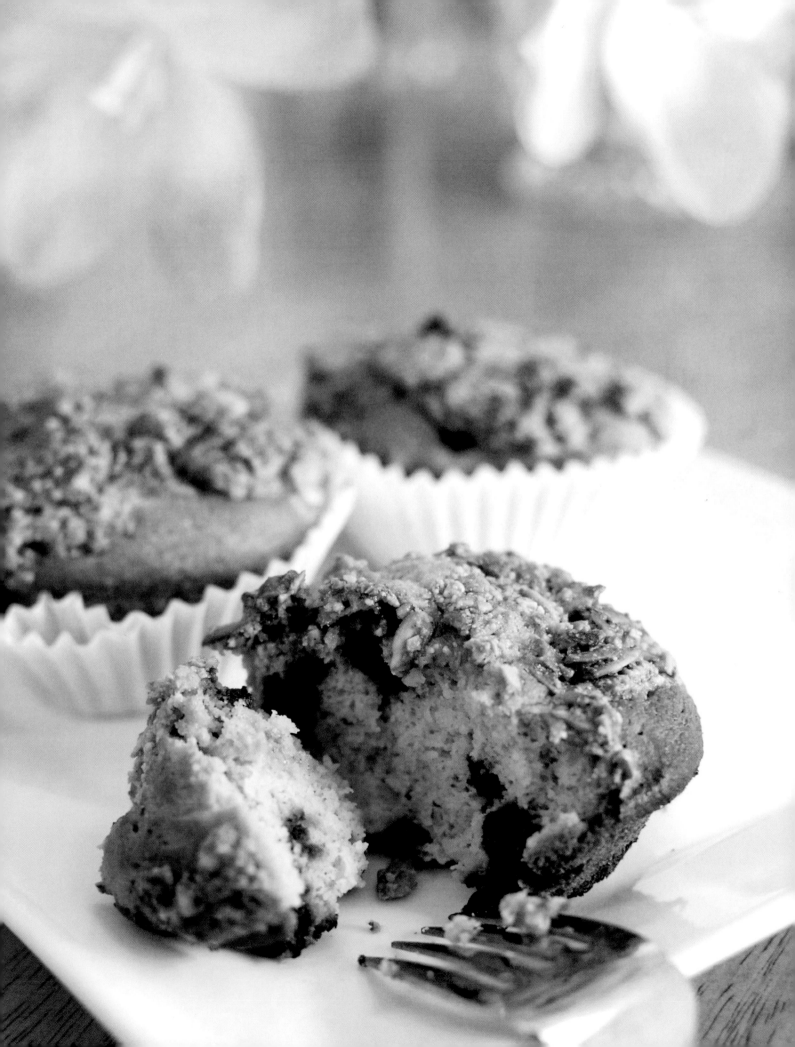

Lemon Poppy Seed Muffins

Makes 6 muffins

Dairy Free • Nut Free • Fish Free

Dry Ingredients

⅓ cup (35 g) coconut flour, sifted

½ tsp baking powder

¼ tsp sea salt

Wet Ingredients

4 eggs

¼ cup (60 mL) pure maple syrup

2 tsp pure vanilla extract

2 TBSP fresh lemon juice (about 1 lemon)

2 tsp lemon zest (about 1 lemon)

¼ cup (60 mL) coconut oil, melted

Add In

2 tsp poppy seeds

Lemon is one of my favorite flavors, almost tied with chocolate—almost. So every once in a while, when I miss the comforting aroma and flavor of a good lemon poppy seed bread, these little muffins really hit the spot. Light and airy, with that slight tanginess from fresh lemons, these muffins really make a rainy spring morning seem light and bright.

1. Preheat the oven to 350°F.

2. Place the dry ingredients in a medium bowl and whisk to combine.

3. Add the wet ingredients, except the coconut oil, and blend well with a hand mixer.

4. With the mixer on low, slowly pour in the coconut oil. Blend well.

5. Stir in the poppy seeds.

6. Fill 6 paper-lined muffin cups two-thirds full with batter.

7. Bake 21-25 minutes, or until golden brown on top and the center of each muffin springs back when pressed lightly.

8. Cool 5-10 minutes in the pan. Serve! Store any leftovers in an airtight container up to 3 days, or freeze up to 3 months.

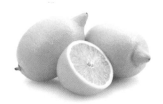

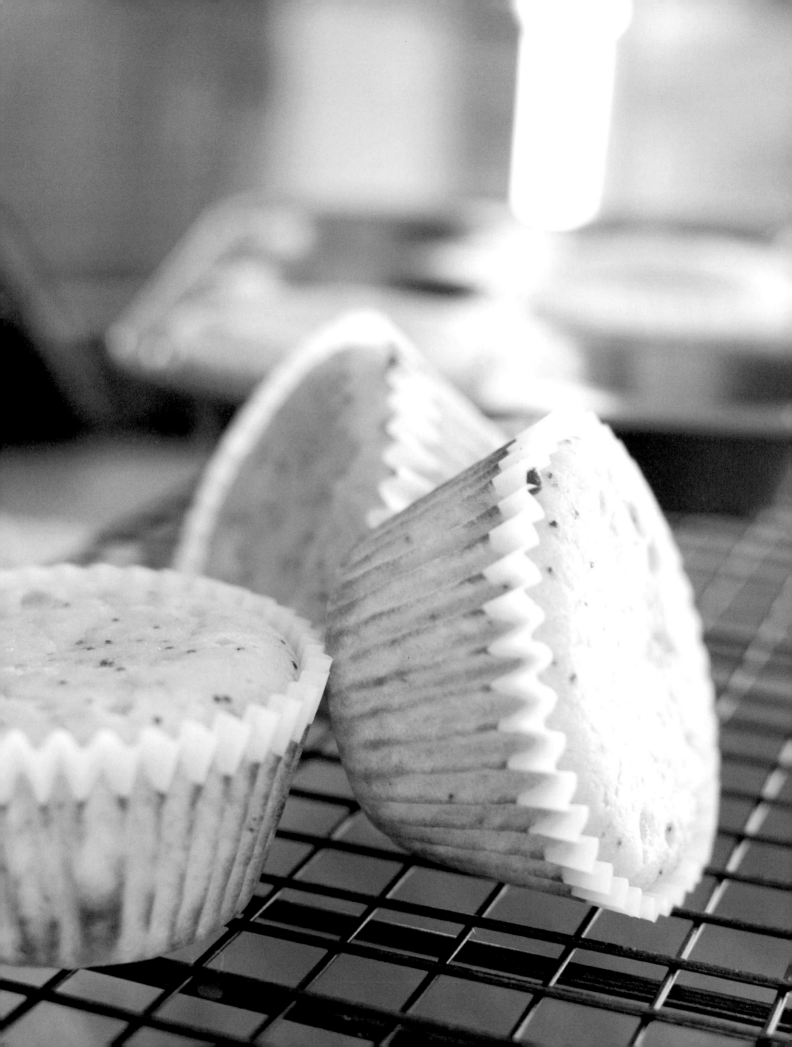

Cinnamon-Swirl Rolls

Makes 8 rolls

Dairy Free • Fish Free

Yeast Mixture

¼ cup (60 mL) warm water

2 tsp raw honey

2 rounded tsp active dry yeast

Dry Ingredients

¾ cup (65 g) almond flour

3 TBSP coconut flour, sifted

⅓ cup (40 g) arrowroot starch

Pinch sea salt

Wet Ingredients

2 eggs

2 TBSP pure maple syrup

1 TBSP coconut oil, melted

Filling

¼ cup (60 mL) coconut oil, melted

Cinnamon

Coconut crystals

So some of you might get a little excited at seeing yeast in a Paleo book. Well, yeast is one of those gray-area items: you don't want to eat it all the time, but every once in a while it's fine, if you can tolerate it. I included this recipe because I, along with many, many people I've talked with, love and miss the taste of a good yeast bread. Sure, I can get a fluffy bread with strictly Paleo ingredients, but yeast provides a taste and texture like nothing else. This is one of those recipes that I make only on rare occasions. These aren't meant for everyday consumption, but if you're about to dash out to your local bakery to down something loaded with gluten and sugar, these rolls are your best, delicious defense.

1. Preheat the oven to 350°F.

2. Place the yeast ingredients in a small bowl and mix together. Set aside until foamy, about 5 minutes.

3. Place the dry ingredients in a medium bowl and whisk to combine.

4. Add the yeast mixture and the wet ingredients to the dry and blend well with a hand mixer.

5. Let the dough rest 5 minutes.

6. Place the dough on a parchment-lined baking sheet and spread with a rubber spatula into the shape of a rectangle, about ⅜-inch thick.

7. Bake 8-9 minutes.

8. Remove pan from the oven.

9. For the filling: Pour the coconut oil over the top, then sprinkle with plenty of cinnamon and some coconut crystals.

10. Carefully (pan is hot) pick up one of the long ends of the parchment paper and start rolling the dough onto itself forming one long "roll." Then, using the parchment paper, slide the cinnamon-roll log back to the center of the pan.

11. Return to the oven and bake 20 minutes more, or until the top is golden brown and a toothpick inserted in the center comes out clean.

12. Place tray on a wire rack and cool 5 minutes before cutting into 8 individual rolls and serve!

13. Delicious alone or with a dab of Vanilla Frosting (page 62).

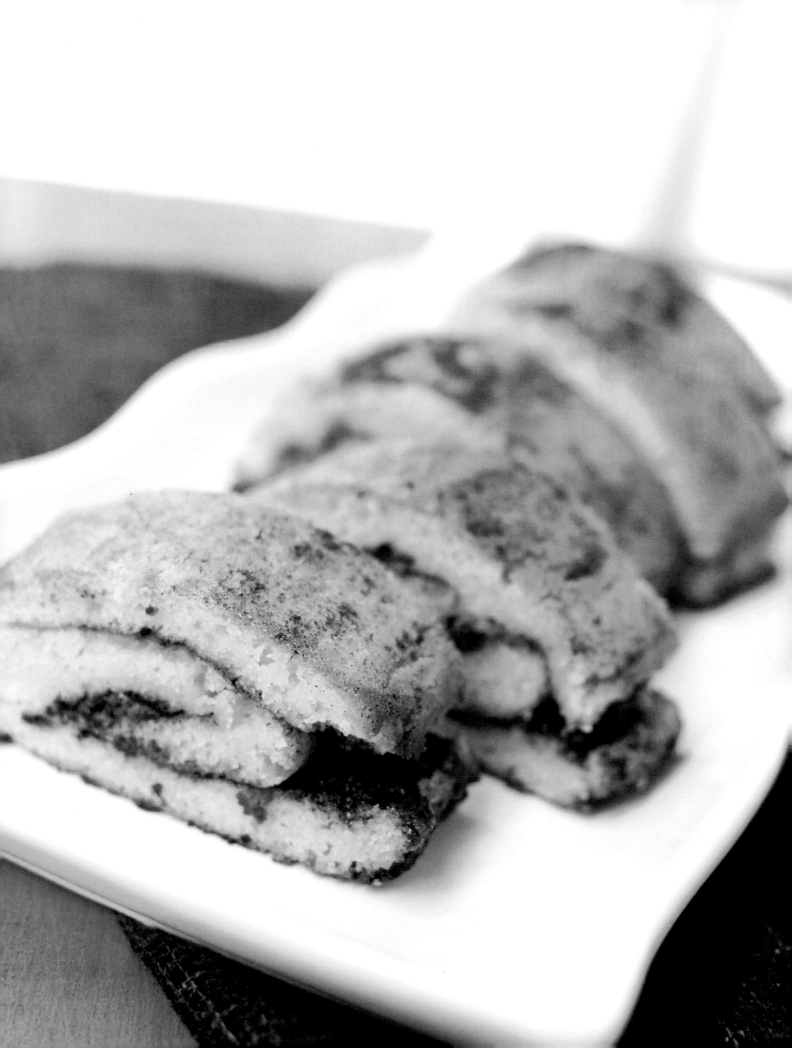

Super-Quick Bread

Makes 1 single-serving loaf
Dairy Free • Fish Free

Dry Ingredients

⅓ cup (40 g) almond flour

1 TBSP coconut flour, sifted

½ tsp baking powder

Pinch sea salt

Wet Ingredients

2 TBSP coconut oil, melted
(plus 1 tsp extra for greasing
the cup)

1 egg

2-3 TBSP water, if needed

I have a freezer full of homemade, sugar-free jams that have been taunting me lately. I needed a vessel to share the glory of this wonderful homemade goodness. That's how this bread came about. There are a few versions floating around the Internet, but most were too nutty tasting from almond flour or had the texture of a cooked egg. I like the balance of almond flour, coconut flour and egg in this version. Slightly toasted it makes a great accomplice for my homemade jam!

1. Place the dry ingredients in a small bowl and stir to combine.

2. Place 1 teaspoon melted coconut oil in a 2-cup glass measuring cup (or large coffee mug) and swirl it around to coat the sides.

3. Add the egg and remaining 2 tablespoons coconut oil to the dry ingredients. Mix well with a fork. If the batter is too thick, add 1 tablespoon of water at a time until it reaches a thick muffin batter consistency.

4. Pour the batter into the measuring cup.

5. Place cup in the microwave and cook on high heat for 1 minute 20 seconds to 1 minute 45 seconds, depending on your microwave.

6. Let the "loaf" cool for 1 minute in the cup, then invert it onto a plate, tapping the bottom of the cup if necessary to get it to release.

7. Serve!

Note:
This bread is great toasted. Simply let it cool for a few minutes, slice it in half, and then place in your toaster oven!

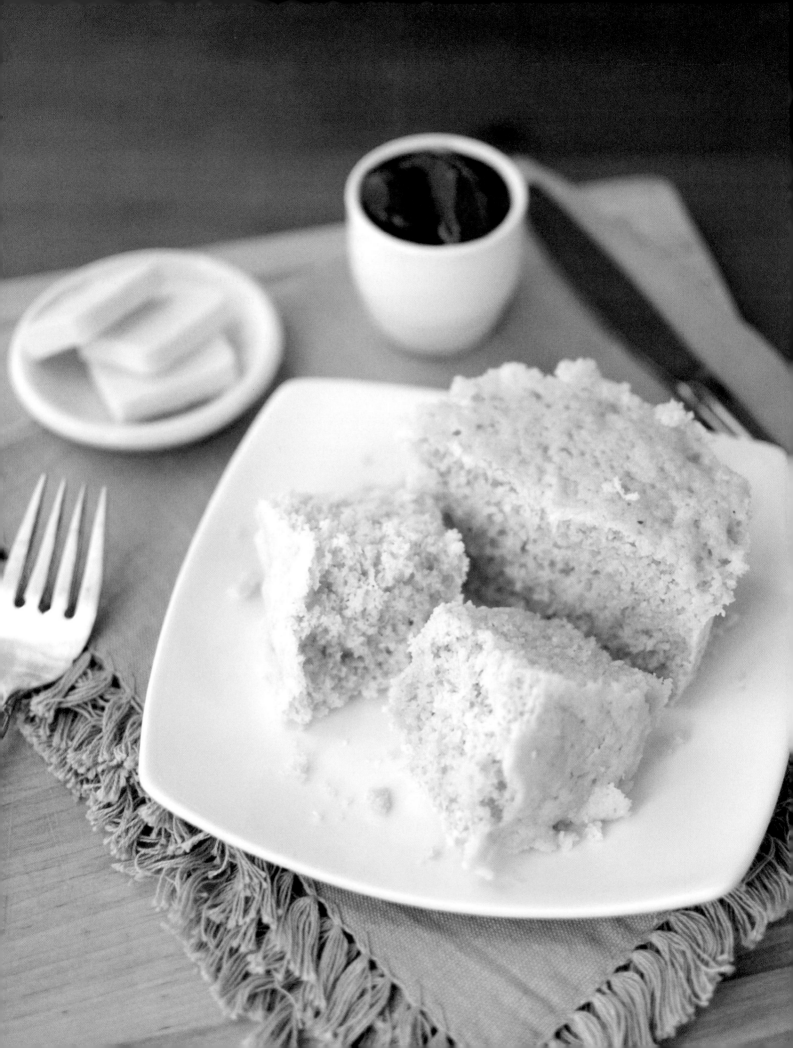

Orange Olive Oil Bread

Makes 2 mini loaves

Dairy Free • Fish Free

Dry Ingredients

⅓ cup (35 g) coconut flour, sifted

⅓ cup (40 g) hazelnut flour (I use Bob's Red Mill)

½ tsp baking soda

¼ tsp sea salt

Wet Ingredients

5 eggs

⅓ cup (80 mL) pure maple syrup

¼ cup (60 mL) extra-virgin olive oil

2 tsp pure vanilla extract

Zest and juice from 1 medium orange

I first made a gluten-free version of this bread that was a huge hit with my family and with clients. When we transitioned into a Paleo lifestyle, I wanted to see if I could capture the same flavor without all the grains and added sugar. Well, it was such a success that it disappeared from my kitchen counter in minutes! The fragrant olive oil moistens this bread like nobody's business, and it combines beautifully with the sweet orange. You might want to double this recipe!

1. Preheat the oven to 350°F.

2. Place the dry ingredients in a medium bowl and whisk to combine.

3. Add the wet ingredients to the dry and blend well with a hand mixer.

4. Grease 2 mini-loaf pans with cooking spray or palm shortening. Divide the batter evenly between the pans.

5. Bake 33-38 minutes, or until the center of the loaf springs back when lightly pressed.

6. Cool 10 minutes in the pans, then turn out onto a wire rack to cool completely. Slice and serve!

7. Store leftovers in an airtight container up to 3 days, or freeze up to 3 months.

Note:

Try topping with Vanilla Frosting (page 62). Add some orange zest to the frosting first for extra flavor.

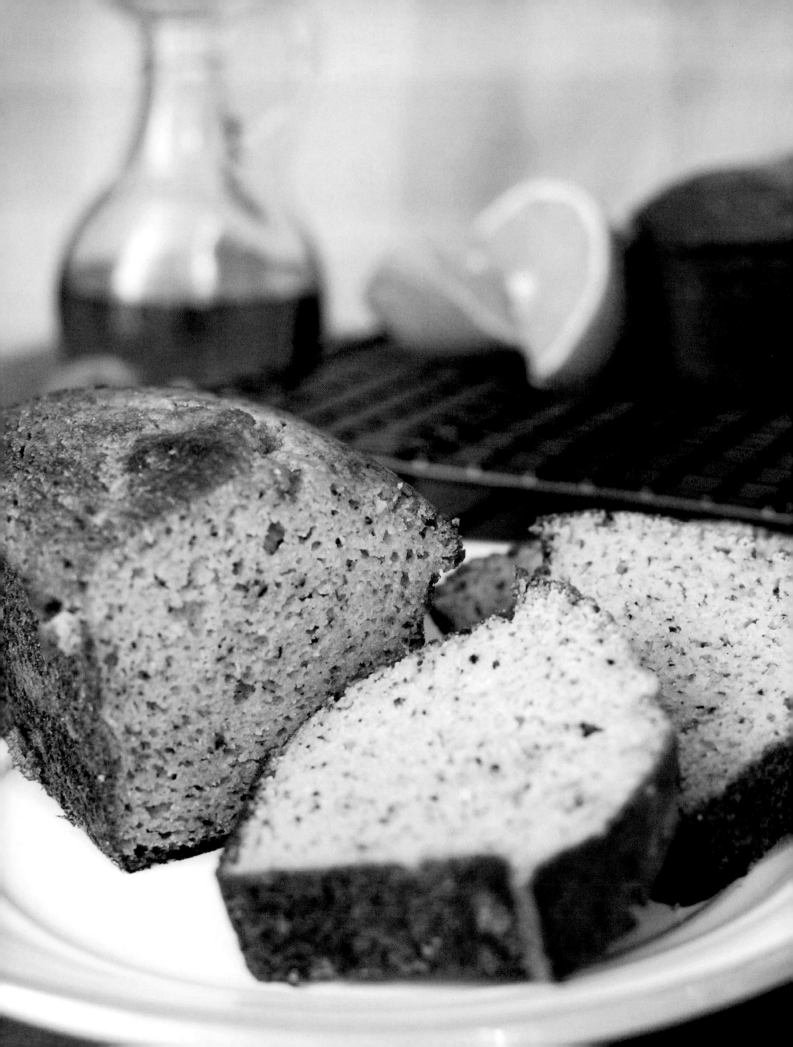

Gingerbread Mini-Loaves

Makes 2 mini loaves
Dairy Free • Nut Free • Fish Free

Dry Ingredients

⅓ cup (35 g) coconut flour, sifted

¼ tsp sea salt

½ tsp baking powder

3 tsp cinnamon

¼ tsp nutmeg

1 tsp ground ginger

Wet Ingredients

4 eggs

2 tsp pure vanilla extract

¼ cup (60 mL) pure maple syrup

¼ cup (60 mL) coconut milk (full-fat or light)

2 TBSP coconut oil, melted

Whether we like it or not, we live in, and have been raised in, a society in which food takes center stage at many special occasions. Because of this, food has an amazingly powerful emotional connection in our lives. This holds true for me, especially during the holidays. I can still smell the wonderful breads and cookies my mom would make during this magical time. And while I don't want to partake in the large amounts of sugar and gluten any longer, these are precious family memories I want to preserve and pass on to my kids. This is where an indulgence like this gingerbread comes into play. It enables me to fill the house with traditional holiday smells, spend some quality bonding time with my kids, and still maintain my nutritional goals. For me, there's nothing healthier than that.

1. Preheat the oven to 350°F.

2. Place the dry ingredients in a medium bowl and whisk to combine.

3. Add the wet ingredients, except the coconut oil, and blend well with a hand mixer.

4. With the mixer on low, slowly add the coconut oil. Blend well. Let batter sit for 5 minutes to thicken.

5. Grease 2 mini-loaf pans with cooking spray or palm shortening. Divide batter evenly between both the pans.

6. Bake 33-38 minutes, or until the center of bread is firm to the touch and a toothpick inserted in the center of the loaf comes out clean.

7. Cool 5 minutes in the pans. Remove loaves from pans and cool completely on wire racks. Frost with Cinnamon-Maple Frosting (page 48) if desired. Store in an airtight container up to 3 days, or freeze up to 3 months.

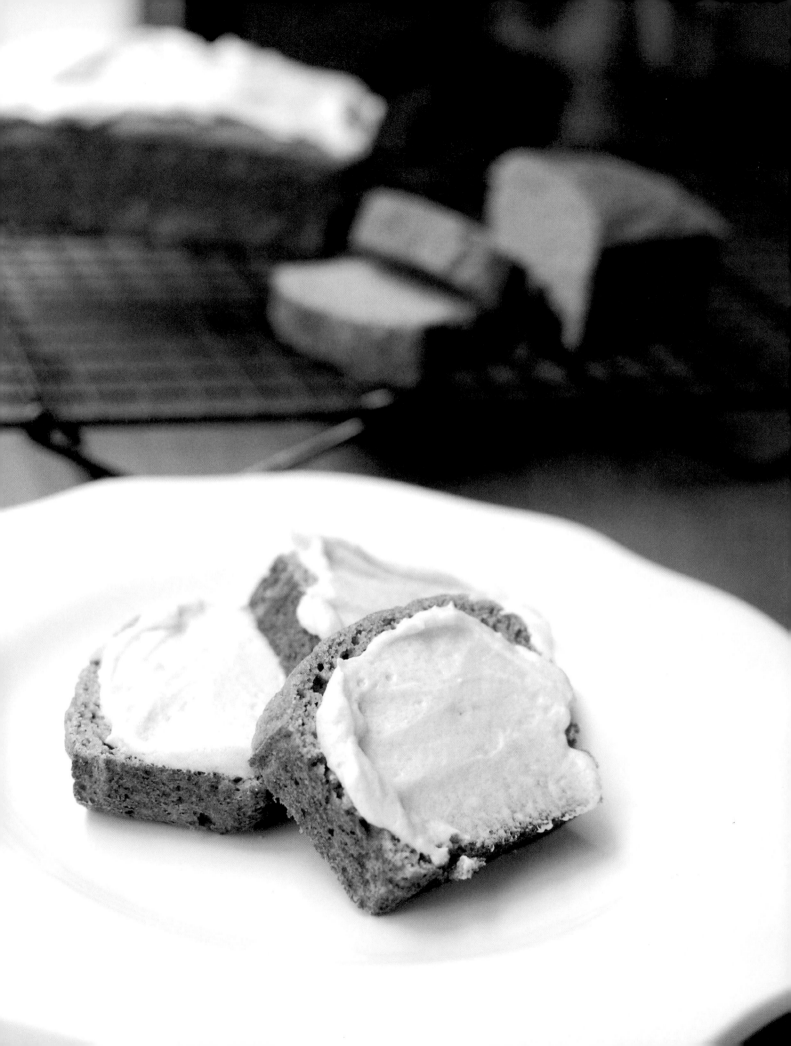

Cinnamon Maple Frosting

Makes 1¼ Cups

Dairy Free • Egg Free • Fish Free • Nut Free

½ cup (95 g) palm shortening

⅓ cup (80 mL) pure maple syrup

Pinch sea salt

1 tsp cinnamon

2 tsp pure vanilla extract

2 TBSP arrowroot starch

2 tsp coconut flour, sifted

2 TBSP coconut oil, melted

I never, ever thought I could love another frosting more than chocolate. I was a dedicated chocolate lover…faithful. But then I whipped up this little number to top my Gingerbread Mini-Loaves (page 46) and I must admit I strayed. Sorry chocolate, but this cinnamon frosting is rich, satisfying and creamy, with that nostalgic punch of cinnamon that just gets me all happy! Enjoy it on gingerbread, Whoopie Pies (page 68) or Vanilla Cupcakes (page 60) and you'll understand my unfaithfulness. Chocolate frosting and I can still be friends though, right?

1. Place all the ingredients, except the coconut oil, in a medium bowl, and use a hand mixer to blend until fully combined.

2. With the mixer on low, slowly add the coconut oil, blending until completely smooth.

3. If frosting is a bit too soft, refrigerate until firm, about 1-2 hours. Blend again to fluff up before using.

4. Frosting can be stored in the refrigerator up to a week. Let it soften a bit at room temperature and fluff it up with a hand mixer before using.

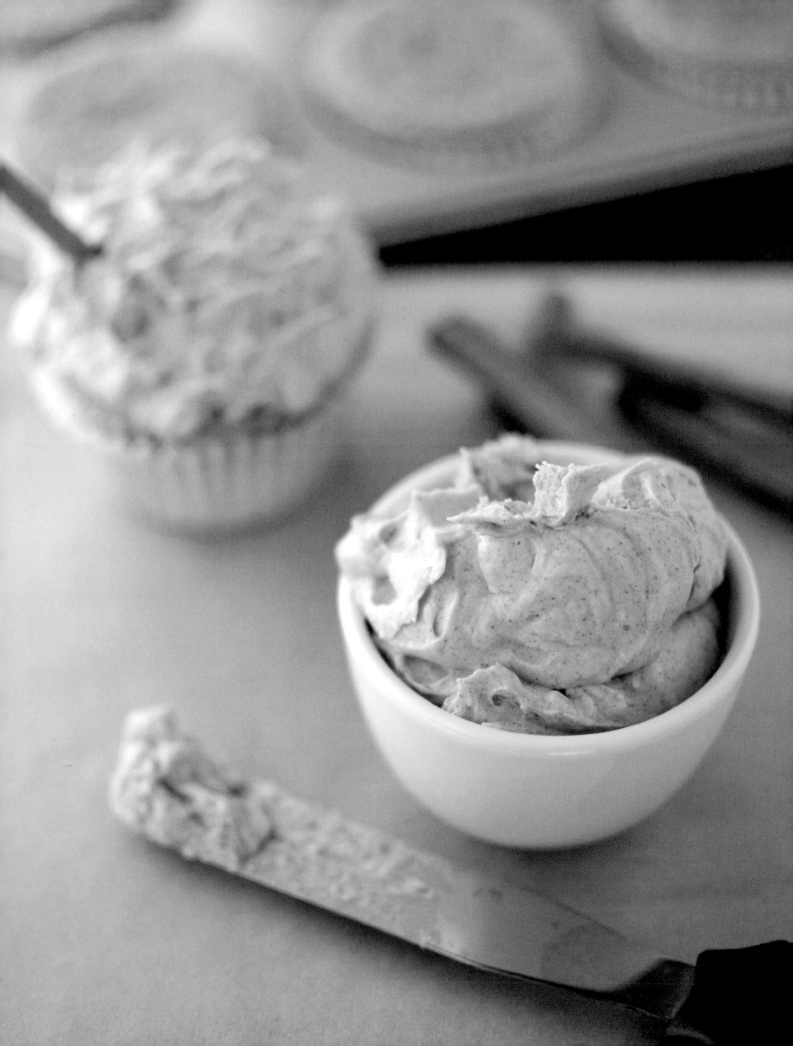

No-Bake Chocolate Tarts

Makes 4 (4-inch) tarts
Dairy Free • Egg Free

Shells

1½ cups (180 g) almond flour

¼ cup (25 g) unsweetened cocoa powder

¼ cup (60 mL) coconut oil, melted

1 TBSP pure maple syrup

Pinch sea salt

Filling

½ cup (120 mL) coconut oil, melted

1 TBSP unsweetened cocoa powder

1 TBSP pure maple syrup

2-3 TBSP full fat coconut milk for a softer filling (optional)

Who would have guessed that so few ingredients could deliver so much satisfying chocolaty goodness?! The combination of almonds, chocolate, maple syrup, and coconut oil works beautifully to create a gourmet dessert with very little effort. No one will believe you didn't slave over an oven for hours—or that it's Paleo! And since you can make these tarts a week ahead, or freeze them, there's no excuse to deprive your guests at your next dinner party or holiday table.

1. Place all the shell ingredients in a medium bowl and mix with a spoon until they start to stick together.

2. Place 1-2 tablespoons of the mixture in each of the 4 mini-tart pans, or, for a less-formal presentation, cupcake liners (I use 3 or 4 together for sturdiness), pressing firmly along the bottom and part way up the sides of the pans. Place on a baking sheet and chill until firm, about 1 hour.

3. Meanwhile, place the filling ingredients in a medium bowl and whisk until smooth.

4. Divide filling evenly between the chilled shells. Refrigerate for another hour, or until filling is firm.

5. Keep refrigerated until ready to serve. Store in an airtight container in the refrigerator up to a week, or in the freezer up to 3 months; simply thaw in the fridge a few hours before serving.

Notes:

Try replacing the almond flour with hazelnut meal, pecan meal, or, for a nut-free version, roasted sunflower seed meal by finely grinding about 2 cups of your preferred nut or seed.

For even more flavor in your filling, try adding ¼ teaspoon pure vanilla, peppermint, or almond extract before mixing it thoroughly.

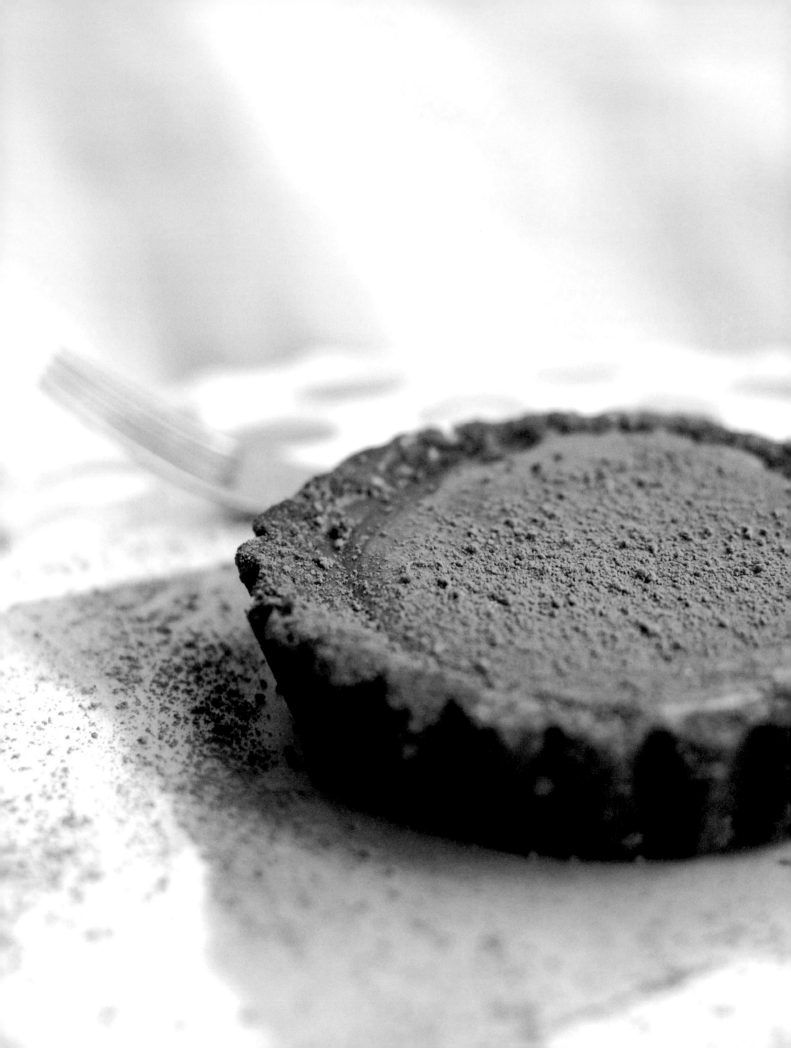

No-Bake Meyer Lemon Tarts

Makes 4 (4-inch) tarts
Dairy Free • Egg Free

Shells

1 cup (120 g) almond flour

⅓ cup (30 g) unsweetened finely shredded coconut

¼ cup (60 mL) coconut oil, melted

1 tsp pure maple syrup

½ tsp pure vanilla extract

Pinch sea salt

Filling

⅓ cup (80 mL) raw cashews, soaked in water overnight

½ cup (120 mL) coconut oil, melted

Juice from 2 Meyer lemons (regular lemons work too)

3 TBSP coconut butter, softened

1 TBSP pure maple syrup

¼ tsp lemon zest (about ½ lemon)

Creating dairy free desserts that are still creamy and decadent can be a challenge. For this recipe I utilized cashew cream; a wonderfully versatile concoction of pureed, soaked raw cashews that gives you a creamy, neutral tasting base for desserts or sauces, without the dairy. Now, I know there's quite a Paleo debate whether cashews are legumes, but you can snack with peace of mind knowing that cashews are indeed not a legume, according to the USDA. So enjoy the lemony, creamy, tangy, sweet goodness of these luscious little tarts all summer long!

1. Place all the shell ingredients in a medium bowl and mix with a spoon until they start to stick together.

2. Place 1 rounded tablespoon of the mixture in each of the 4 mini-tart pans, or cupcake liners (I use 3 or 4 together for sturdiness), pressing firmly along the bottom and part way up the sides of the pans. Place on a baking sheet and chill until firm, about 1 hour.

3. Meanwhile, make the filling. Place the soaked cashews in a food processor and pulse until puréed.

4. Add the remaining filling ingredients and purée until smooth, about 2 minutes.

5. Divide the filling evenly among the chilled shells. Refrigerate for another hour, or until filling is firm.

6. Keep refrigerated until ready to serve. Store in the refrigerator in an airtight container up to a week, or in the freezer up to 3 months: simply thaw in the fridge for a few hours before serving.

Note:

Try replacing the almond flour with hazelnut meal, pecan meal, or, for a nut-free version, raw sunflower seed meal by grinding about 2 cups of your preferred nut or seed.

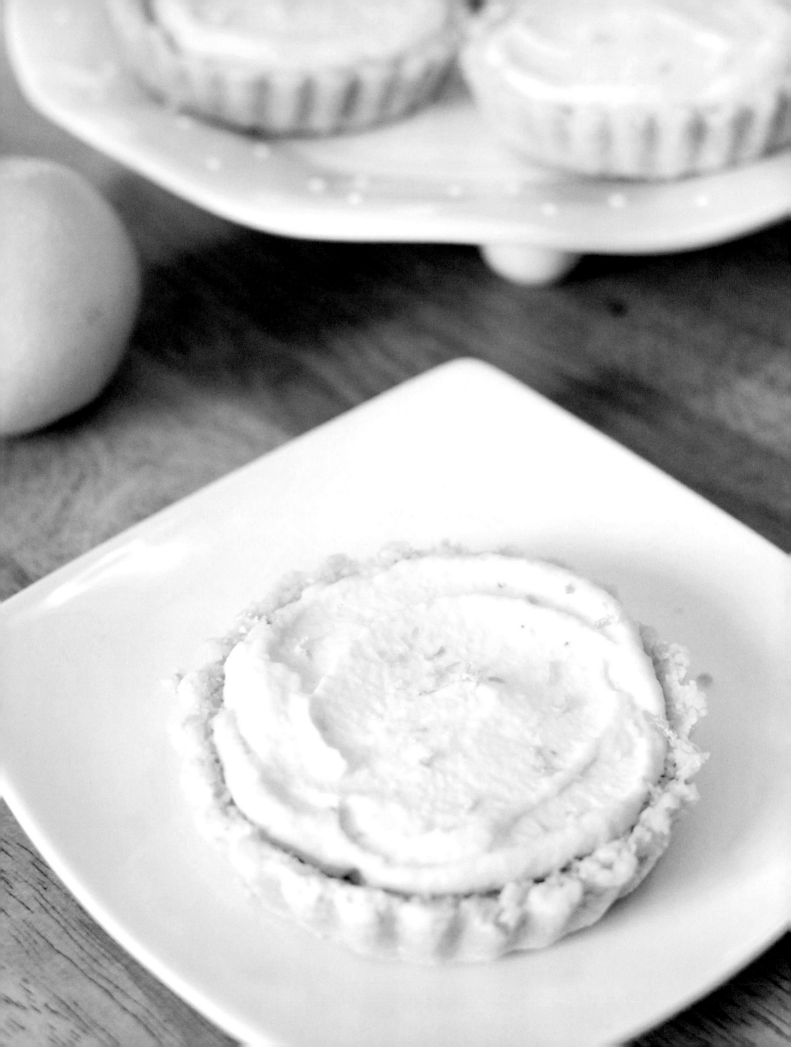

No-Bake Pumpkin Tarts

Makes 8 (4-inch) tarts
Dairy Free • Egg Free • Fish Free

Shells

3 cups (450 g) roasted walnuts or pecans

⅔ cup (60 g) unsweetened, finely shredded coconut

⅔ cup (160 mL) coconut oil, melted

1 TBSP pure maple syrup

2 tsp pure vanilla extract

Pinch sea salt

Filling

1 envelope unflavored gelatin

¼ cup (60 mL) cold water

¾ cup (180 mL) canned pumpkin

⅓ cup (80 mL) pure maple syrup

½ tsp cinnamon

⅛ tsp nutmeg

¾ cup (140 mL) coconut milk (full-fat or light)

1 TBSP pure vanilla extract

Pinch sea salt

Add On

Cinnamon or pumpkin pie spice

Whipped cream or whipped coconut cream

I like this variation on a traditional pumpkin pie for holiday celebrations. Everyone gets an individual dessert, which always puts smiles on faces. Plus, these can be made in advance, so you can enjoy your holiday guests more. Spend more time at your social gathering and less time hunting and gathering with this easy-to-make dessert!

1. Place the walnuts in a food processor and pulse until a fine meal forms.

2. Place the walnut meal and the remaining shell ingredients in a medium bowl and stir to combine.

3. Divide the mixture evenly among 8 mini-tart pans, pressing firmly on the bottom and up the sides. Place in the fridge to firm up.

4. Meanwhile, make the filling. In a small saucepan, sprinkle the gelatin over the cold water and let it soften 1 minute.

5. Turn the heat to medium and bring the mixture just to a simmer, stirring until the gelatin has dissolved. Remove from heat.

6. Whisk in the remaining filling ingredients until well combined.

7. Divide the pumpkin mixture evenly among the tart shells. Place on a baking sheet and chill until set, about 3 hours. Garnish with a sprinkle of cinnamon or pumpkin pie spice and a spoonful of whipped cream or whipped coconut cream.

8. Keep refrigerated until ready to serve. Store in the refrigerator in an airtight container up to 4 days, or in the freezer up to 3 months: simply thaw in the fridge for a few hours before serving.

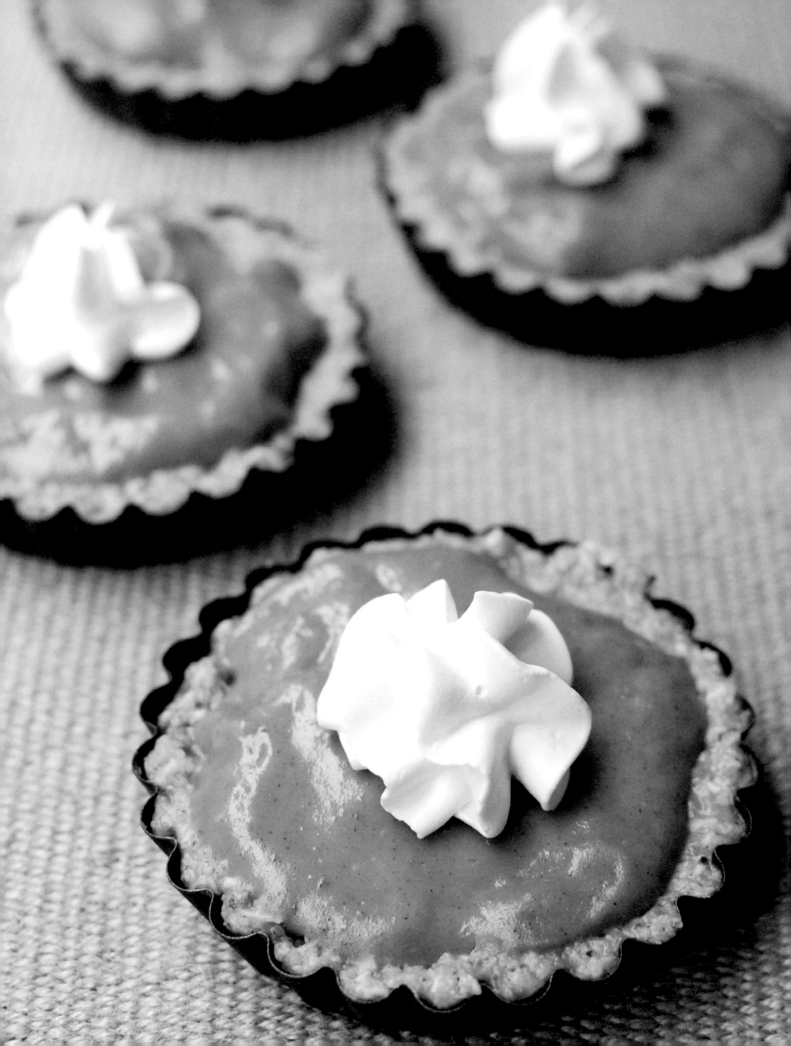

Chocolate Mini-Bundts

Makes 6 cakes

Dairy Free • Fish Free • Nut Free

Dry Ingredients

¼ cup (25 g) coconut flour, sifted

¼ tsp sea salt

½ tsp baking powder

¼ cup (25 g) unsweetened cocoa powder

Wet Ingredients

4 eggs

1 TBSP pure vanilla extract

¼ cup (60 mL) pure maple syrup

¼ cup (60 mL) coconut milk (full-fat or light)

¼ cup (60 mL) coconut oil, melted

The first thing my oldest daughter said to me when I told her about my latest cookbook adventure was, "Mom, it better have chocolate cake in it! You know I love chocolate cake." Well, my lovely daughter, this one's for you! Moist, rich, and fluffy, this recipe can be made as cupcakes or, my favorite, mini-bundts! This one just might keep me in the running for "Mom of the Year!" At least until I forget to pick them up at school one day. Not that I've ever done that.

1. Preheat the oven to 350°F.

2. Place the dry ingredients in a medium bowl and whisk to combine.

3. Add the wet ingredients, except the coconut oil, to the dry and mix well with a hand mixer.

4. With the mixer on low, slowly pour in the coconut oil. Mix well.

5. Divide the batter evenly among a 6-cavity greased mini-bundt pan.

6. Bake 22-25 minutes, or until the center of the cakes spring back when pressed lightly.

7. Cool 10 minutes in the pan and then turn out onto a wire rack. Cool completely before frosting.

8. Frost with Chocolate (page 58), Vanilla (page 62), or Strawberry Frosting (page 64)!

Note:

For cupcakes, bake 22-25 minutes, cool in the pan 5 minutes, then remove and cool completely on a wire rack.

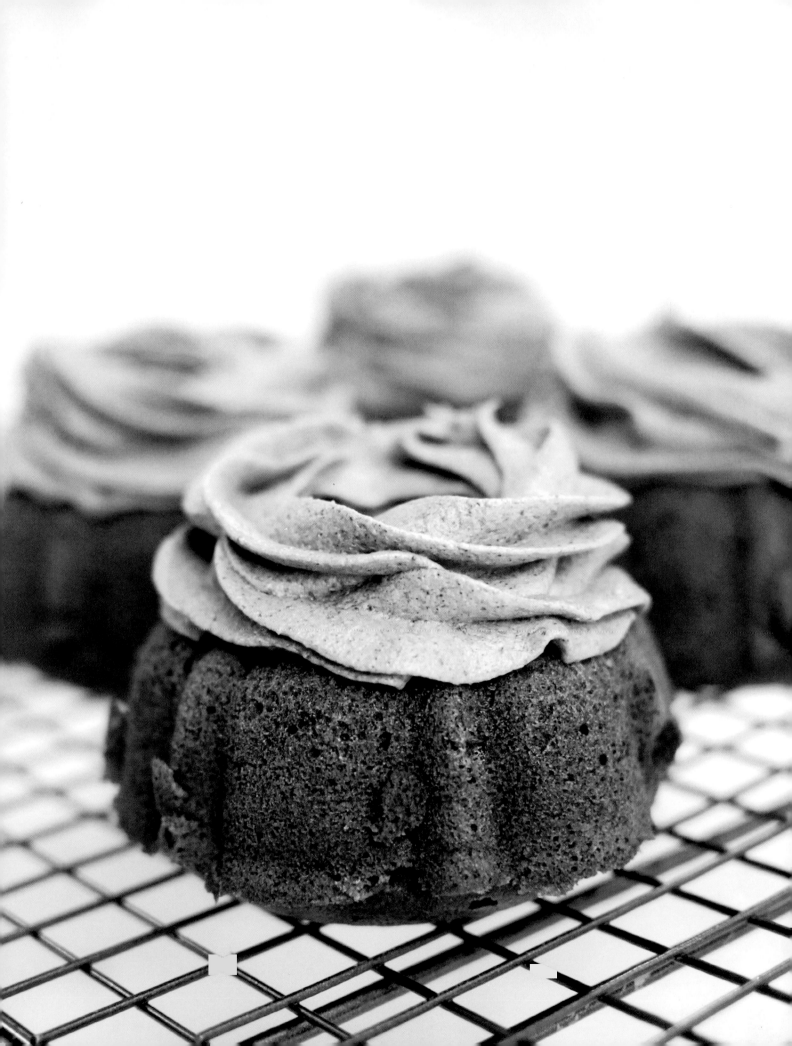

Chocolate Frosting

Makes 1 ¼ Cups

Dairy Free • Egg Free • Fish Free • Nut Free

½ cup (95 g) palm shortening

⅓ cup (80 mL) pure maple syrup

Pinch sea salt

2 tsp pure vanilla extract

2 TBSP arrowroot starch

1 tsp coconut flour, sifted

2 TBSP unsweetened cocoa powder

2 TBSP coconut oil, melted

Finding a sugar-free frosting that can withstand more than 5 minutes out of the refrigerator is tough. But my frostings really hold up well under pressure. Now, they won't last too long in super-high heat, say all day at a midsummer picnic, but they will provide a great birthday treat for someone's special day in normal room-temperature party situations. Just keep them in a cooler if you think your location is too hot to handle.

1. Place the shortening, maple syrup, and salt in a medium bowl, and use a hand mixer to combine.

2. Add the vanilla, arrowroot, coconut flour, and cocoa powder and blend again.

3. With the mixer on low, slowly add the coconut oil until incorporated. Whip frosting on high until light and fluffy.

4. Refrigerate if needed to firm up a bit, and then whip again.

5. Frosting can be stored in the refrigerator up to a week. Let it soften a bit at room temperature and fluff it up with a hand mixer before using.

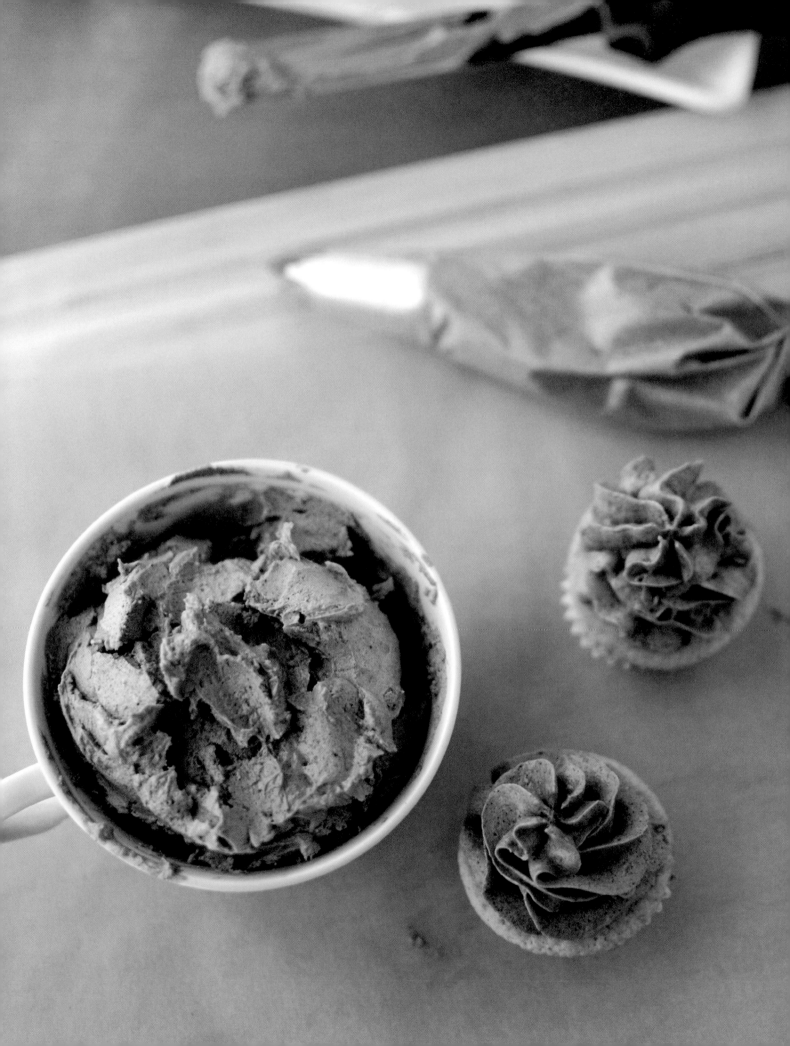

Vanilla Cupcakes

Makes 6 cupcakes
Dairy Free • Fish Free • Nut Free

Dry Ingredients

⅓ cup (35 g) coconut flour, sifted

¼ tsp sea salt

½ tsp baking powder

Wet Ingredients

4 eggs

1 TBSP pure vanilla extract

¼ cup (60 mL) pure maple syrup

¼ cup (60 mL) coconut milk (full-fat or light)

½ vanilla bean, split and scraped (optional)

¼ cup (60 mL) coconut oil, melted

Every special birthday needs a special treat, and these are my youngest daughter's favorite birthday cupcakes! Because they're so light, soft, and delicious, no party guest has ever figured out they weren't the real thing. I won't tell if you won't!

1. Preheat the oven to 350°F.

2. Place the dry ingredients in a medium bowl and whisk to combine.

3. Add the wet ingredients, except the coconut oil, to the dry and mix well with a hand mixer.

4. With the mixer on low, slowly pour in the coconut oil. Mix well.

5. Divide the batter among 6 paper-lined muffin cups.

6. Bake 22-25 minutes, or until the center of the cupcakes spring back when pressed lightly in the center.

7. Cool in the pan 5 minutes, then turn out onto a wire rack. Cool completely before frosting.

8. Frost with Chocolate (page 58), Vanilla (page 62) or Strawberry Frosting (page 64)!

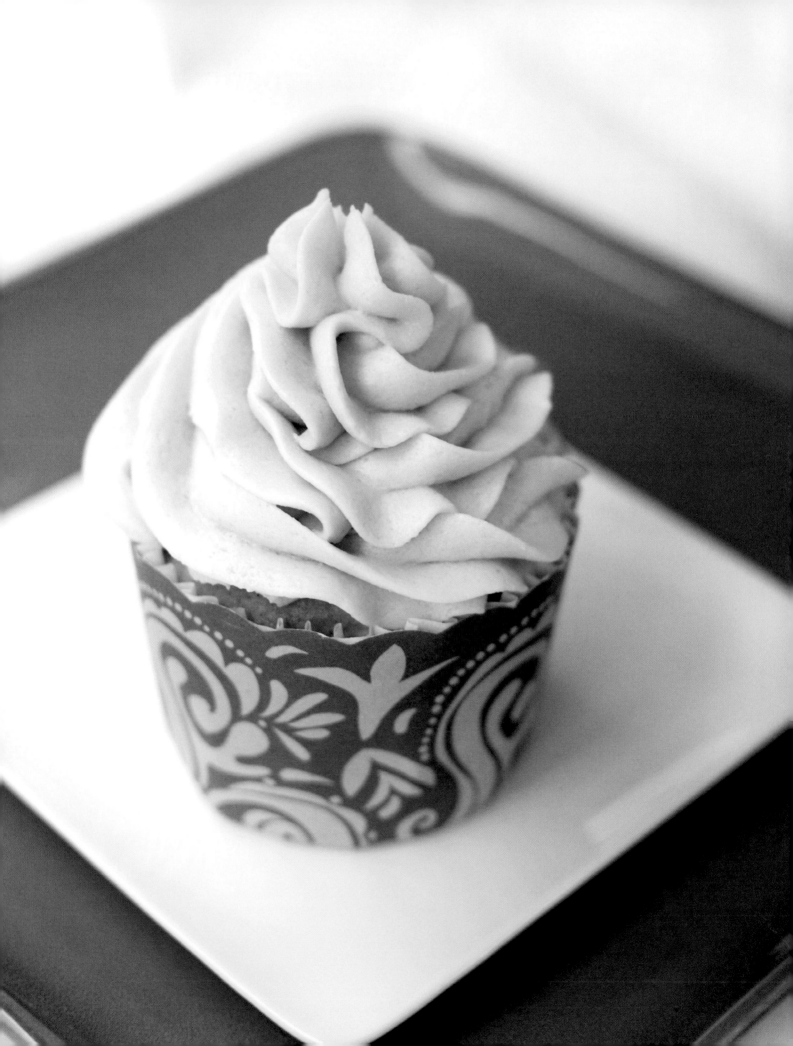

Vanilla Frosting

Makes 1 ¼ Cups
Dairy Free • Egg Free • Fish Free • Nut Free

½ cup (95 g) palm shortening

⅓ cup (80 mL) pure maple syrup

2 tsp pure vanilla extract

2 TBSP arrowroot starch

2 tsp coconut flour, sifted

Pinch sea salt

2 TBSP coconut oil, melted

This frosting is so creamy, rich, and satisfying, you'll never guess it's free of powdered sugar and butter. Best of all, it's super-versatile: use it to ice Cinnamon-Swirl Rolls (page 40), to top Orange Olive Oil Bread (page 44), or sandwich it between Whoopie Pies (page 68) for a classic dessert. I love food that multitasks!

1. Place all the ingredients, except the coconut oil, in a medium bowl, and use a hand mixer to blend until fully combined.

2. With the mixer on low, slowly add the coconut oil, blending until completely smooth.

3. Frosting can be stored in the refrigerator up to a week. Let it soften a bit at room temperature and fluff it up with a hand mixer before using.

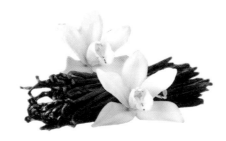

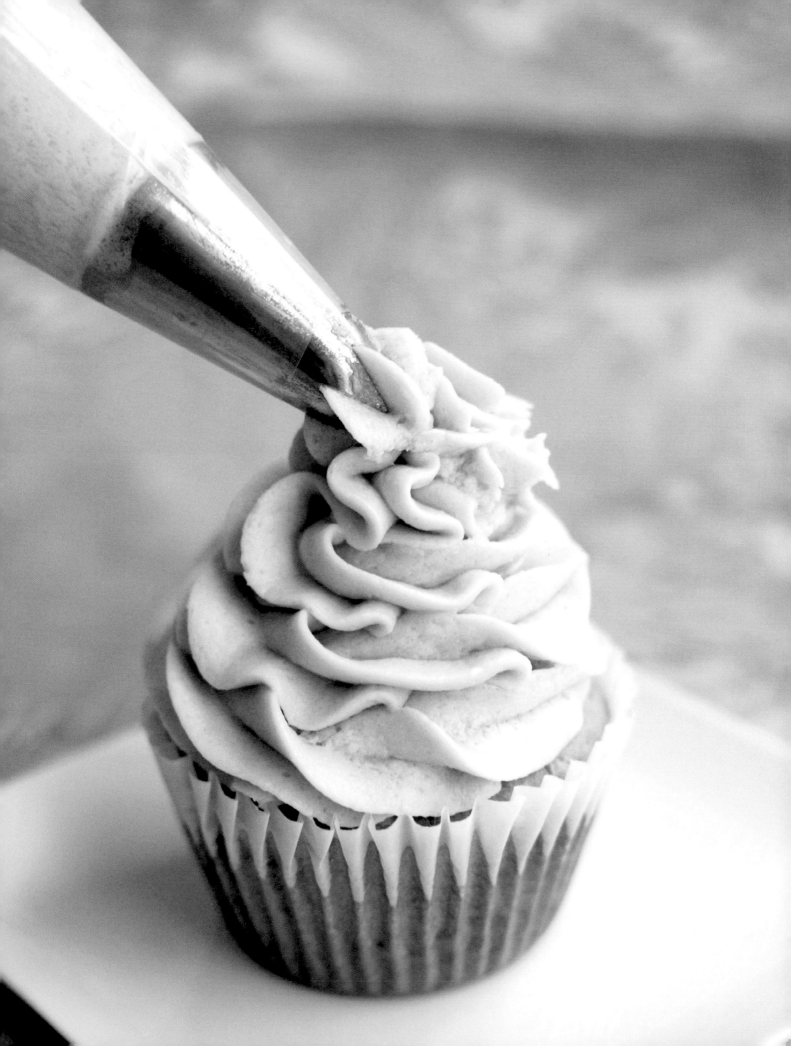

Strawberry Frosting

Makes 1 ¼ Cups

Dairy Free • Egg Free • Fish Free • Nut Free

1 cup (34 g) unsweetened, unsulfured freeze-dried strawberries

½ cup (95 g) palm shortening

⅓ cup (80 mL) pure maple syrup

2 tsp pure vanilla extract

2 TBSP arrowroot starch

2 tsp coconut flour, sifted

Pinch sea salt

2 TBSP coconut oil, melted

I've recently discovered the wonderful versatility and overall yumminess of unsweetened, unsulfured freeze-dried fruit! Delicious in trail mix, or—my favorite—ground into a powder and added to all sorts of goodies, like this frosting, freeze-dried fruits can help you add a powerful punch of concentrated flavor without an excessive amount of sugar.

1. Place the strawberries in a food processor and process until they turn into powder.

2. Place the strawberry powder and remaining ingredients, except the coconut oil, in a medium bowl, and use a hand mixer to blend until fully combined.

3. With the mixer on low, slowly add the coconut oil, blending until completely smooth.

4. Frosting can be stored in the refrigerator up to a week. Let it soften a bit at room temperature and fluff it up with a hand mixer before using.

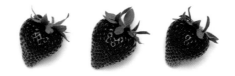

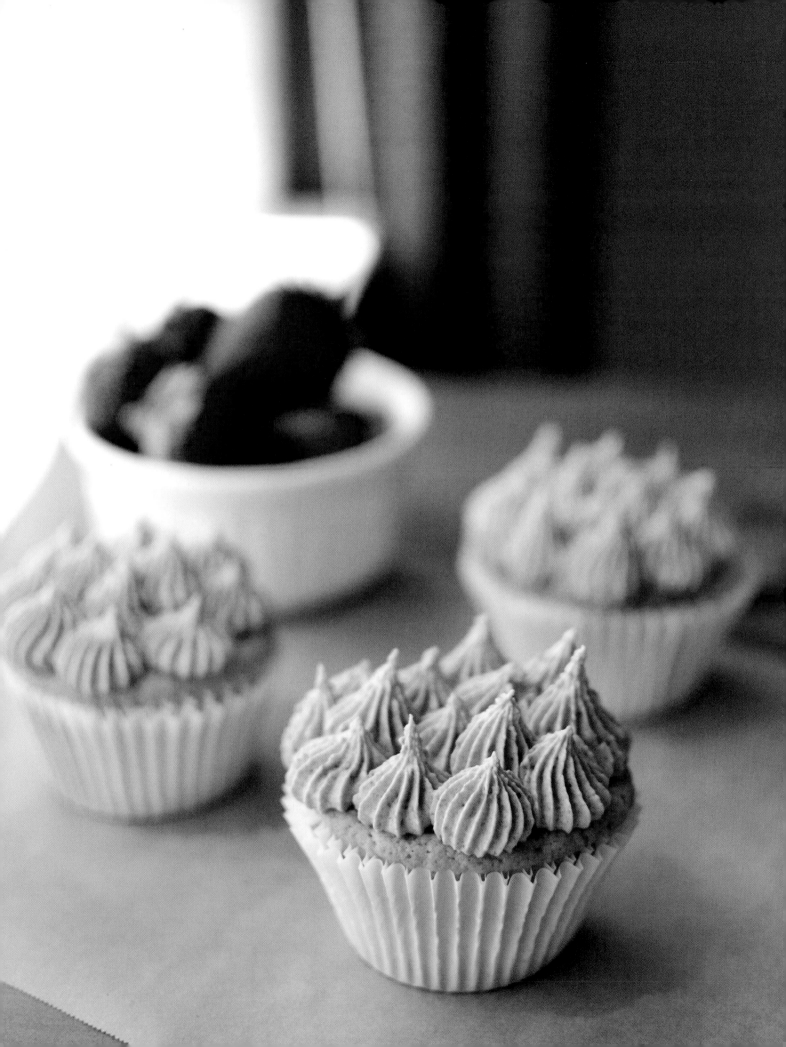

One-Minute Chocolate Cake

Enough for 2 to share

Dairy Free • Fish Free

Dry Ingredients

3 TBSP almond flour

2 tsp coconut flour, sifted

1 TBSP flax meal (freshly ground golden flaxseeds)

½ tsp baking powder

1½ TBSP unsweetened cocoa powder

Pinch sea salt

Wet Ingredients

2 TBSP coconut oil

3 TBSP pure maple syrup

1 egg

1 tsp pure vanilla extract

Topping

Chocolate Frosting (page 58)

I love living a Paleo lifestyle because I don't have the intense multiple-times-per-day sugar cravings I did before. I feel more in control of the food I consume, and therefore find it easier to be more mindful when I have the occasional treat. Those who still eat the standard American diet full of grains and sugar find it hard to believe that these cravings subside. I know I doubted it. And the icing on the cake, as they say, is that when I do indulge, a little sweetness goes a long way: I don't have to make a giant batch of cookies and eat them for days on end. A small taste and I'm good for a while. This cake is perfect for that reason. Easy, healthy, and with no leftovers to keep tempting you, it'll satisfy your occasional chocolate craving, without knocking you off the Paleo wagon.

1. Place the dry ingredients in a small bowl and whisk to combine.

2. Melt the coconut oil in a 2-cup glass measuring cup or large mug. Pour most of the coconut oil into the dry ingredients, leaving a small amount in the cup to grease the bottom and up the sides.

3. Add the remaining wet ingredients to the bowl. Mix well.

4. Pour into the greased measuring cup. Microwave on high for 1 minute 30 seconds to 1 minute 45 seconds.

5. Let cake cool 1-2 minutes in the cup. Place a small serving plate over the cup, then turn it over to release the cake. Cool just until slightly warm. Frost and enjoy!

Note:

For a quick go-to icing, combine 2 tablespoons dark chocolate and ½ teaspoon palm shortening in a microwave safe bowl. Heat in the microwave for 20 second increments, until almost completely melted, stirring each time. Stir until smooth. Pour over the top of your warm cake!

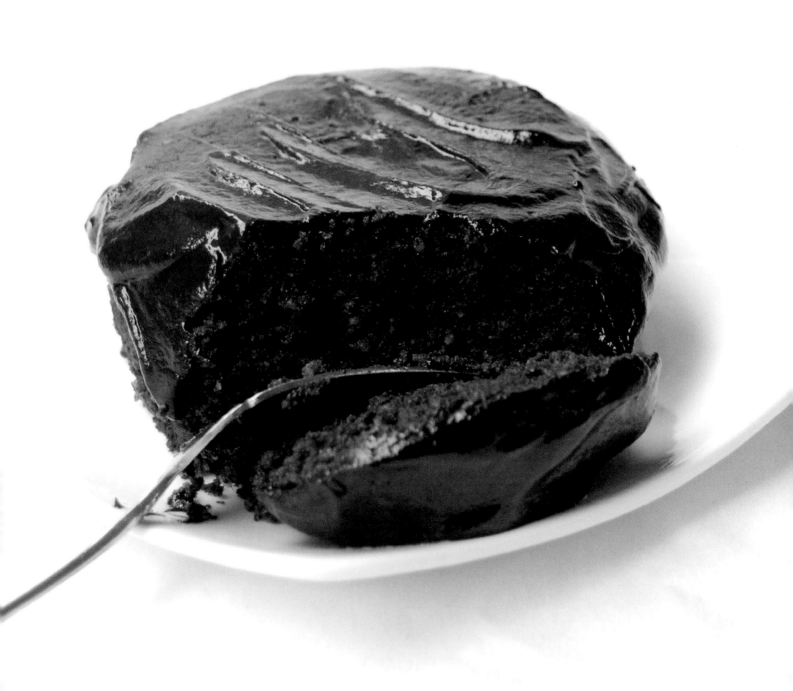

Whoopie Pies

Makes 4 pies
Dairy Free • Fish Free

Dry Ingredients

¼ cup (30 g) almond flour

¼ cup (25 g) coconut flour, sifted

¼ tsp sea salt

½ tsp baking soda

¼ cup (25 g) unsweetened cocoa powder

Wet Ingredients

3 eggs

1 tsp pure vanilla extract

¼ cup (60 mL) pure maple syrup

3 TBSP coconut oil, melted

Filling

Vanilla Frosting (page 62)

I love the regional ties we have with food. My husband, who is originally from the East Coast, adores Whoopie Pies and couldn't wait for me to create a Paleo version. Being from the West Coast, I had no idea what a Whoopie Pie was since we generally called a cake sandwich with a cream filling a Suzy Q. Whatever you want to call these treats, you'll enjoy the combination of soft, chocolaty cake and a creamy vanilla center!

1. Preheat the oven to 350°F.

2. Place the dry ingredients in a medium bowl and whisk to combine.

3. Add the wet ingredients, except the coconut oil, and blend with a hand mixer until combined.

4. With the mixer on low, slowly pour in the coconut oil. Mix well. Let batter sit 5 minutes to thicken.

5. With an ice-cream size scoop, place 8 even mounds of batter on a parchment-lined baking sheet. Flatten and smooth just slightly with a rubber spatula. They will spread a bit when baking.

6. Bake 14-16 minutes, or until firm and the center springs back when pressed lightly.

7. Cool on a wire rack.

8. Place 4 cooled cakes flat side up on a serving tray. Spread Vanilla Frosting on each cake. Top with a second cake (flat side down on top of frosting) and press lightly to stick together. Store leftovers in an airtight container in the fridge up to 3 days, or in the freezer up to 3 months.

Note:
Try using Strawberry Frosting (page 64) or Chocolate Frosting (page 58) in the center for a tasty twist!

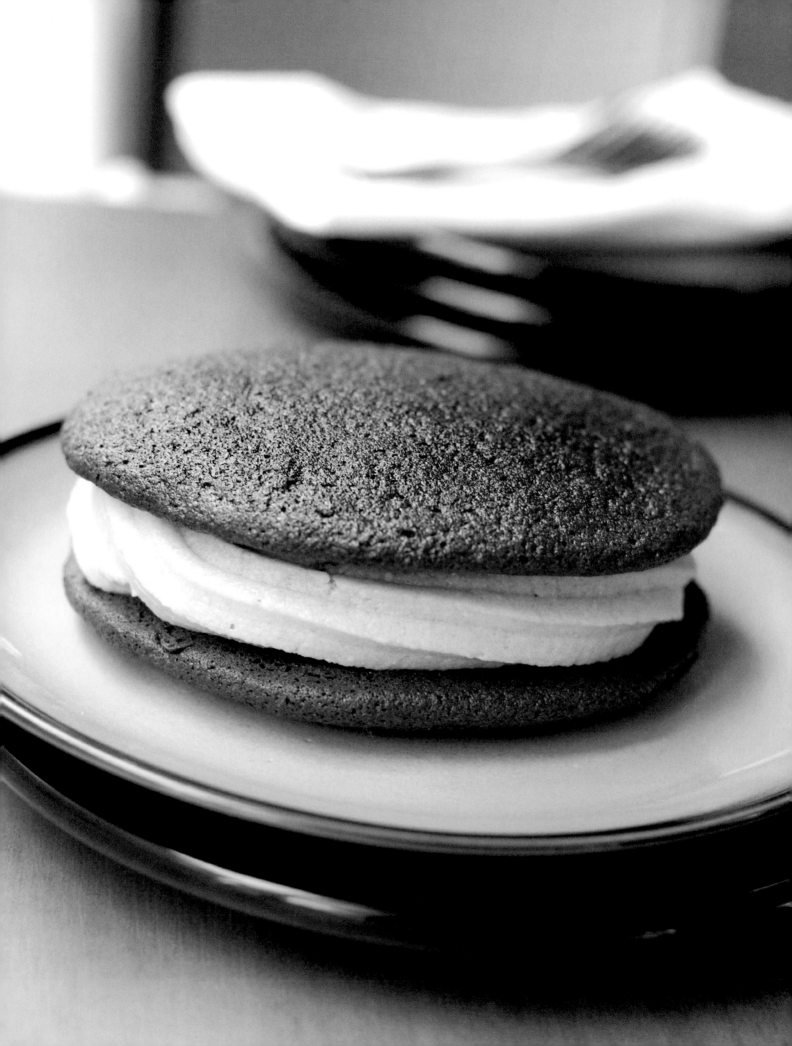

Hazelnut Chocolate Chunk Cookies

Makes about 12 cookies

Dairy Free • Fish Free

Dry Ingredients

2¼ cups (270 g) hazelnut flour (I use Bob's Red Mill)

2 TBSP arrowroot starch

¾ tsp baking soda

Pinch sea salt

Wet Ingredients

2 eggs

2 tsp pure vanilla extract

⅓ cup (80 mL) pure maple syrup

¼ cup (60 mL) coconut oil, melted

Add In

½ cup (80 g) dark chocolate chunks (Enjoy Life brand or chop your own)

I love the combination of fragrant hazelnuts with the dark chocolate in these cookies. It's not your typical almond flour cookie, but rather unique and incredibly satisfying. I love that they stay soft for days and freeze well too! So feel free to make a double batch and keep leftovers in the freezer for a quick grab-and-go indulgence.

1. Preheat the oven to 350°F.

2. Place the dry ingredients in a medium bowl and whisk to combine.

3. Add the wet ingredients, except the coconut oil, to the dry and blend well with a hand mixer.

4. With the mixer on low, slowly pour in the coconut oil. Blend well.

5. Stir in the chocolate chunks.

6. Drop rounded tablespoons of dough onto a parchment-lined baking sheet.

7. Bake 10-12 minutes, or until edges are browned and center is set.

8. Let cookies cool on the tray for 5 minutes. Remove cookies to a wire rack to cool completely. Store in an airtight container up to 3 days, or in the freezer up to 3 months.

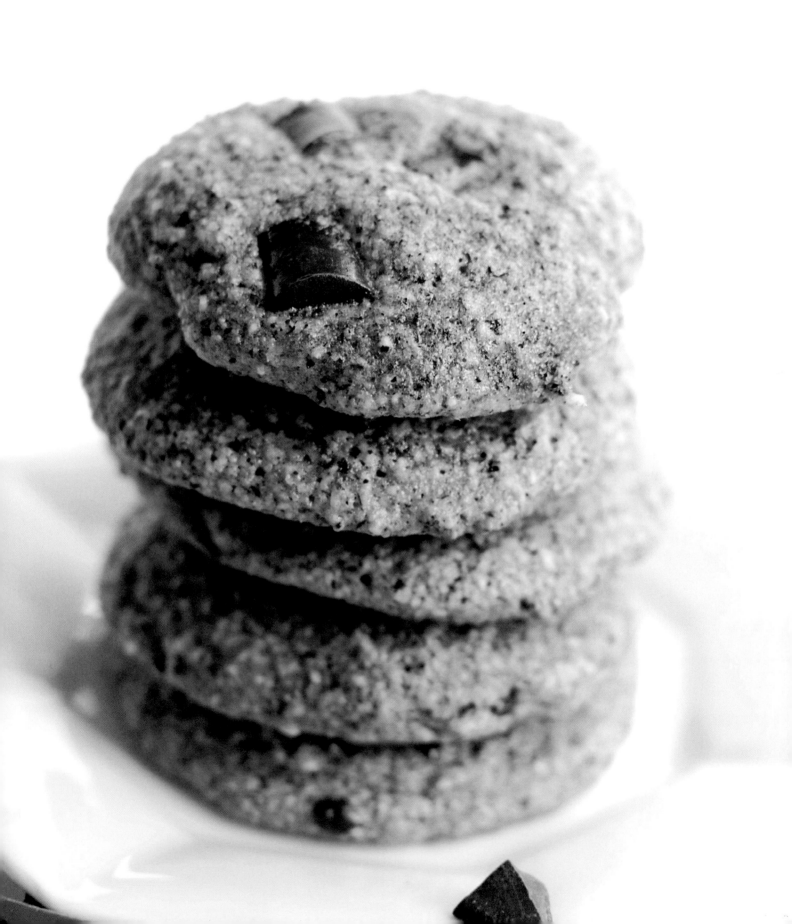

Macadamia-Date Macaroons

Makes about 14 cookies

Dairy Free • Fish Free

8 dates, pits removed, chopped

¾ cup (65 g) unsweetened coconut flakes

¾ cup (110 g) roasted, salted macadamias

½ tsp pure vanilla extract

1 TBSP raw honey

1 egg

With only a handful of ingredients, these macaroon-esque cookies couldn't be simpler. The dates provide plenty of sweetness, and the macadamias add satisfying fat and crunch. They're pretty perfect as-is, but they also provide a blank canvas to let your imagination go crazy: try a few dark chocolate chunks, cinnamon, raisins, or any of your favorite cookie add-ins and see how many varieties you can dream up!

1. Preheat the oven to 350°F.

2. Place all the ingredients in a food processor and pulse until coarsely chopped. You want a slightly chunky consistency, not a smooth paste.

3. Drop rounded tablespoons of dough onto parchment-lined baking sheets.

4. Bake 12-15 minutes, until golden brown on tops and bottoms.

5. Cool on trays placed on wire racks. Store in an airtight container 3-4 days, or freeze up to 3 months.

Note:

If you're using dates that are a little older, use a few extra to help with moisture, or simply soak in warm water for 5 minutes, then drain prior to using.

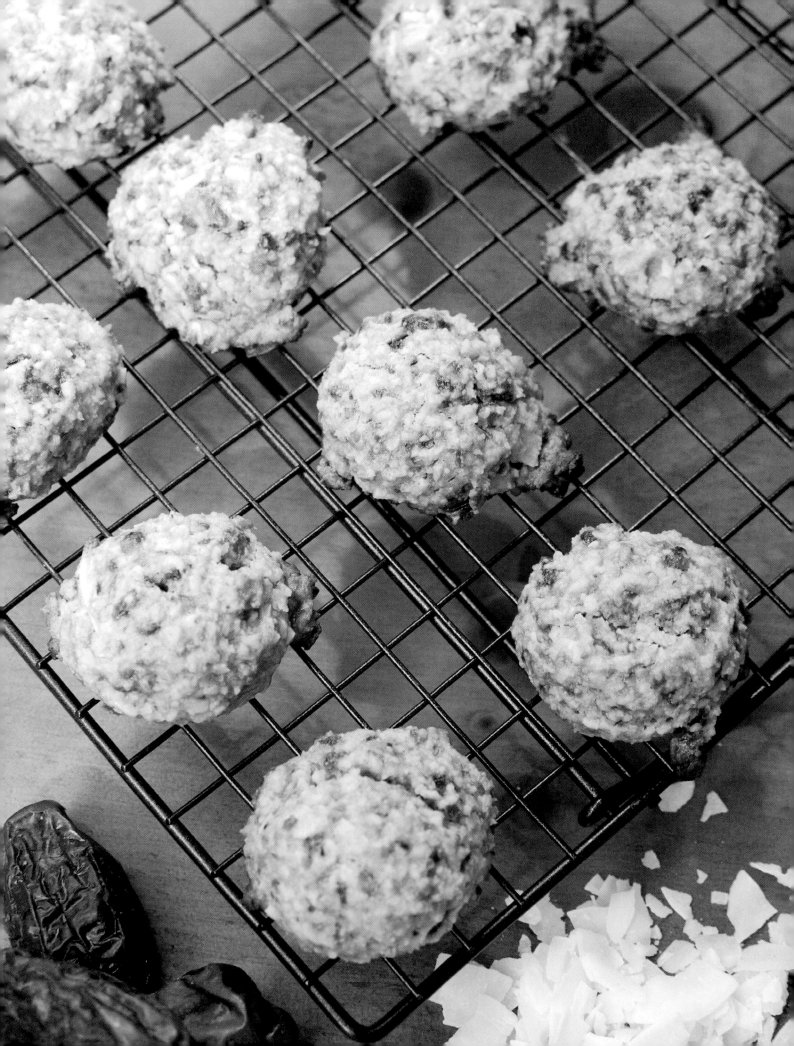

Skinny-Mint Cookies

Makes about 60 cookies
Dairy Free • Fish Free

Dry Ingredients

1¼ cups (150 g) almond flour

½ cup (50 g) coconut flour, sifted

2 TBSP arrowroot starch

¼ cup (25 g) unsweetened cocoa powder

¼ tsp sea salt

Wet Ingredients

½ cup (120 mL) pure maple syrup

1 egg

½ tsp pure peppermint extract

¼ cup (60 mL) coconut oil, melted

Coating

¾ cup (120 g) chopped dark chocolate

2 oz (56 g) unsweetened dark chocolate (100% cacao)

½ tsp pure peppermint extract

Yep, we're talking those minty delights that the girls in uniform deliver every spring—and by far my favorite recipe in this book. Mimicking the texture of those crispy-good cookies from my past was a challenge, but I am oh so happy with the results! So each spring, when your friends are going into a sugar coma from buying too many boxes of "those" cookies, you can make your own! Without an ounce of guilt. Or a headache. Or a stomach ache. You get the picture.

1. Place the dry ingredients in a medium bowl and whisk to combine.

2. Add the wet ingredients, except the coconut oil, to the dry. Blend with a hand mixer.

3. With the mixer on low, slowly pour in the coconut oil. Mix well.

4. Place the dough on a large sheet of plastic wrap. Using the plastic wrap as a guide, shape the dough into a 1¾-inch diameter log. (You can divide the dough into thirds to make it easier.) Wrap tightly and freeze until very firm, about 2 hours.

5. Preheat the oven to 350°F.

6. Remove dough from the freezer and slice into ¼-inch-thick rounds.

7. Place the rounds on 2 parchment-lined baking sheets. Bake 12-14 minutes, or until centers are firm to the touch and the edges start to brown slightly.

8. Remove cookies from trays and cool completely on wire racks.

9. Meanwhile, melt the coating ingredients in the top of a double boiler over simmering water, stirring until smooth.

10. Using 2 forks, dip each cookie in the chocolate coating, scraping off any excess along the edge of the bowl.

11. Return cookies to the parchment-lined baking sheets. Refrigerate until chocolate sets, about 30 minutes to 1 hour. Store cookies in an airtight container in the fridge up to 5 days, or in the freezer up to 3 months.

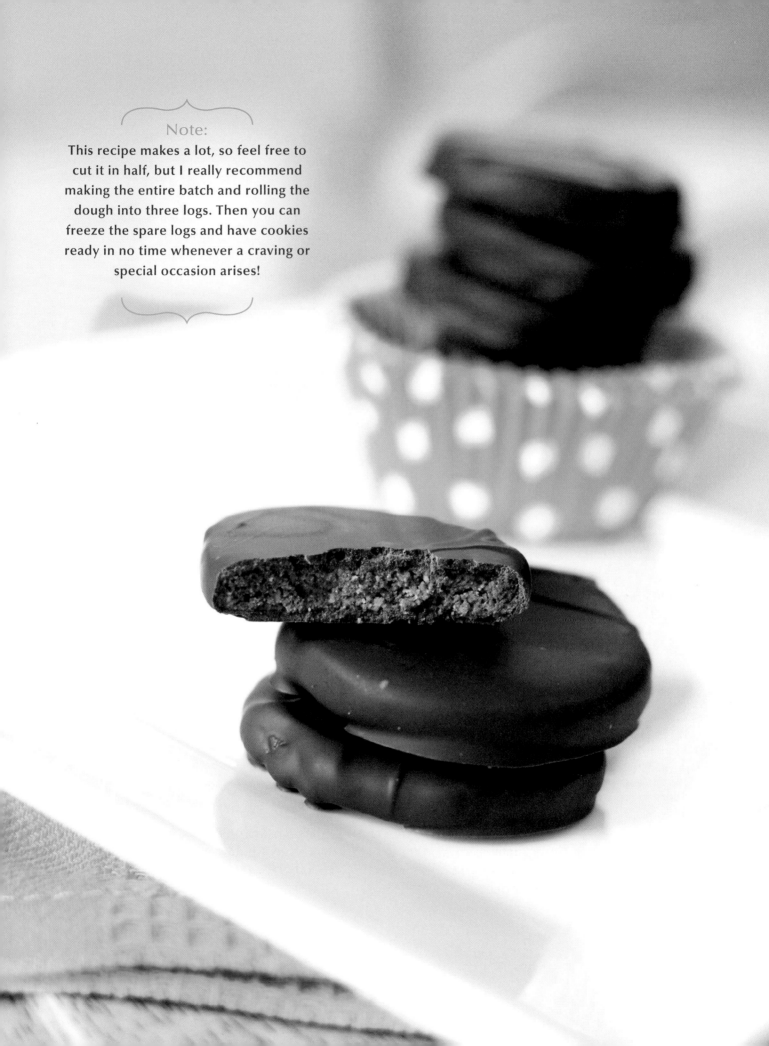

Note:

This recipe makes a lot, so feel free to
cut it in half, but I really recommend
making the entire batch and rolling the
dough into three logs. Then you can
freeze the spare logs and have cookies
ready in no time whenever a craving or
special occasion arises!

Sugar Cookies

Makes 12 large cookies
Dairy Free • Fish Free

Dry Ingredients

1 cup (120 g) almond flour

¼ cup (25 g) coconut flour, sifted

2 TBSP arrowroot starch, plus extra for dusting

½ tsp baking soda

⅛ tsp sea salt

Wet Ingredients

1 egg

2 tsp pure vanilla extract

¼ tsp pure almond extract

⅓ cup (80 mL) pure maple syrup

2 TBSP coconut oil, melted

A classic cookie with a Paleo twist! Worthy of any holiday gift tray, they deliver all the classic sugar cookie scrumptiousness without the classic refined sugar and grains. My kids love making these at Christmas because they know Santa needs a healthy treat after all the gluten and sugar he gets during the rest of his busy night! The dough can take a little getting used to because it is soft, but you'll get the hang of it in no time: just make sure to roll it out between two sheets of parchment paper, cut the shapes, then remove the excess dough!

1. Preheat the oven to 350°F.

2. Place the dry ingredients in a medium bowl and whisk to combine.

3. Add the wet ingredients, except the coconut oil, to the dry and blend with a hand mixer.

4. With the mixer on low, slowly add the coconut oil and mix well.

5. For a soft cookie, you can drop rounded tablespoons of dough onto two parchment lined baking sheets and bake 11-13 minutes.

   • For a crispier cookie, place the dough on plastic wrap and roll into a log. Place in the freezer for 2 hours. Remove and slice into ¼-inch-thick slices. Place on a parchment-lined baking sheet and bake 13-15 minutes or until center is firm to the touch and edges are golden brown.

   • For cutouts, shape dough into a disc and refrigerate 3 hours. Using a fine dusting of arrowroot starch to prevent sticking, dust 2 sheets of parchment paper and the dough. Roll dough out to ¼-inch thickness between two sheets of parchment paper. Remove top sheet of parchment paper and use cookie cutters to cut out desired shapes. Remove excess dough. Place parchment with cookies on a baking sheet and bake 13-15 minutes, or until edges are browned and centers are firm to the touch.

6. Cool cookies on the trays for 5 minutes, then transfer to a wire rack to cool completely. Store in an airtight container up to 5 days, or in the freezer up to 3 months.

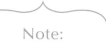

Note:
For a traditional sugar cookie crunch,
you can sprinkle some coconut crystals
on the tops before baking. For a holiday
treat, frost with Chocolate Frosting
(page 58), Vanilla Frosting (page 62) or
Strawberry Frosting (page 64)!

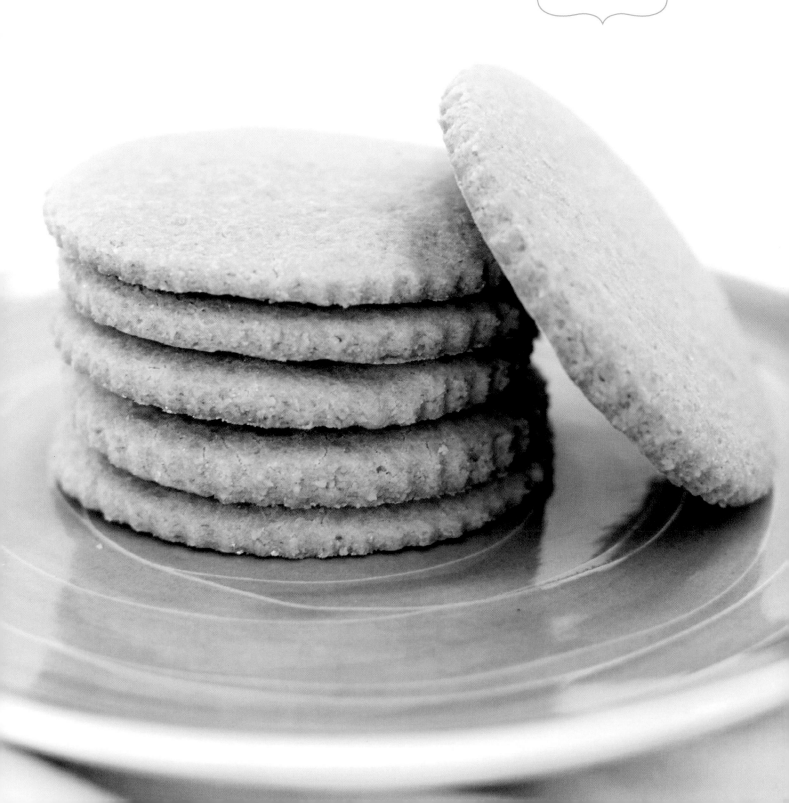

Chocolate-Hazelnut Thumbprints

Makes 8 cookies

Dairy Free • Fish Free

Dry Ingredients

1 cup (120 g) hazelnut flour (I use Bob's Red Mill)

½ cup (50 g) coconut flour, sifted

¼ cup (25 g) unsweetened cocoa powder

½ tsp baking soda

Wet Ingredients

⅓ cup (80 mL) pure maple syrup

1 egg

2 TBSP coconut oil, melted

Filling

2 oz (56 g) dark chocolate, chopped

⅓ cup (80 g) almond butter

3 TBSP coconut oil

Oh, the power of Nutella! You can't view a blog or Pinterest page without seeing a recipe using this popular chocolate hazelnut spread. It really has taken on a life of its own, with good reason, as the flavor combination is quite addictive. But, given that sugar is the first ingredient, followed shortly by soy lecithin and artificial flavors, I think I'll pass on that fad. Instead, try making a batch of these delectable cookies to satisfy that sweet tooth! Made with nutritious hazelnut and coconut flours, these little thumbprints are filling and delicious, without the hype.

1. Preheat the oven to 350°F.

2. Place the dry ingredients in a medium bowl and stir to combine.

3. Add the wet ingredients and mix well with a hand mixer.

4. Drop rounded tablespoons of dough onto a parchment-lined baking sheet. Push your thumb into the top of each cookie, making a well.

5. Bake 10-12 minutes, or until firm on the edges. Cool cookies on trays for 5 minutes, then transfer to a wire rack to cool completely.

6. Meanwhile, make the filling. Place the filling ingredients in a small saucepan over low heat just until melted. Whisk until combined and smooth. Let filling cool and firm up a bit, about 1 hour in the fridge, or until it becomes the consistency of soft butter.

7. Place 1 rounded teaspoon of filling in each cookie. Store in an airtight container in the fridge up to 3 days, or in the freezer up to 3 months.

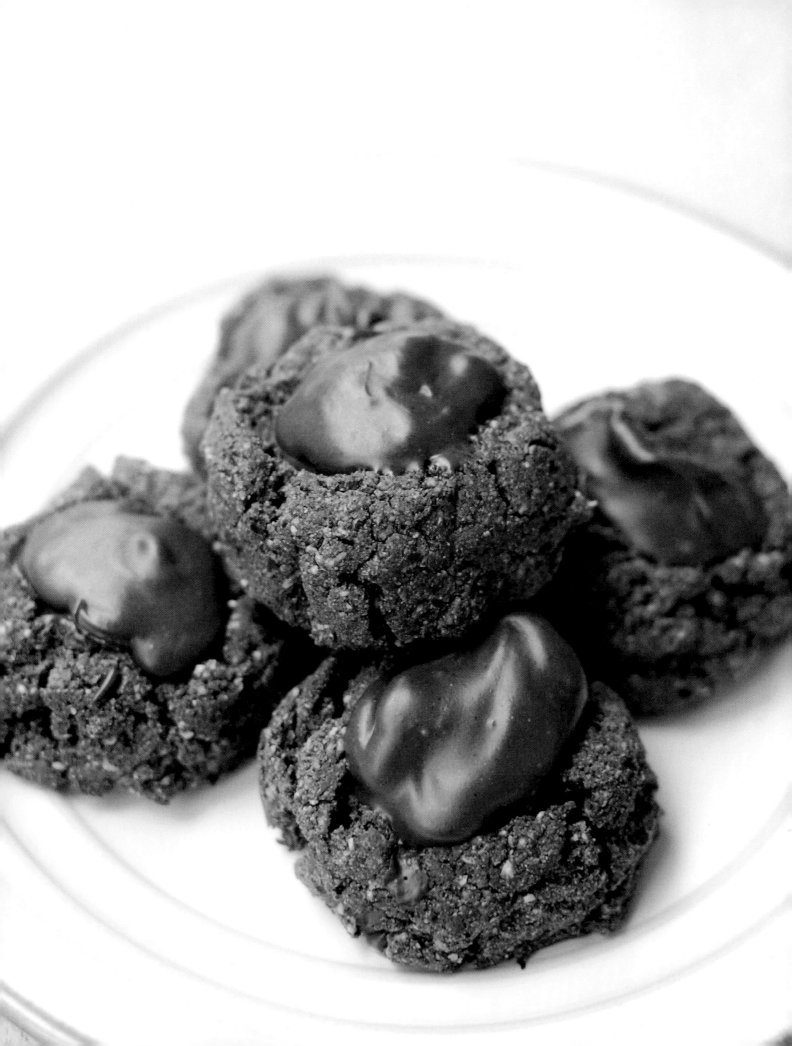

Some-More-Ahhhhhs

Makes 12 cookies

Dairy Free* • Fish Free

For the Cookie

Dry Ingredients

2 cups (240 g) almond flour

½ cup (45 g) unsweetened, finely shredded coconut

½ tsp baking soda

Wet Ingredients

¼ cup (60 mL) pure maple syrup

2 tsp pure vanilla extract

1 egg

3 TBSP coconut oil, melted

For the Caramel

1 cup (200 g) coconut crystals

¼ cup (60 mL) coconut nectar

½ cup (120 mL) full-fat coconut milk

⅓ cup (80 g) butter (*optional)

For the Tops

½ cup (45 g) unsweetened finely shredded coconut

½ cup (80 g) chopped dark chocolate

1 oz unsweetened dark chocolate (100% cacao), chopped

I loved the taste and texture of the coconut-caramel cookies the Girl Scouts would sell each year, but of course, the ingredients list left a lot to be desired. I can't even imagine biting into one of those sugar-bombs these days, but I still wanted to create a cookie with a similar flavor. This soft, coconut-y, caramel-y piece of heaven was just what I envisioned. I must warn you though: They are chewy and delicious, making it tough to eat just one. So make a batch, enjoy one, and then freeze the rest for later!

1. Preheat the oven to 350°F.

2. Make the cookies. Place the dry ingredients in a medium bowl and whisk to combine.

3. Add the wet ingredients to the dry and blend well with a hand mixer. Cover and refrigerate dough 15 minutes.

4. Scoop rounded tablespoonfuls of dough onto two parchment-lined baking sheets. Place six cookies on each tray, as they will spread a little.

5. Bake 12-13 minutes, or until golden brown. Cool cookies on trays for 5 minutes, then transfer to a wire rack to cool completely.

6. Lower oven heat to 300°F.

7. Meanwhile, make the caramel. Place the caramel ingredients in a medium saucepan and stir to combine.

8. Heat over medium-high heat, boiling until mixtures reaches 250°F on a candy thermometer (about 20 minutes).

9. Remove from the heat and let cool about 10 minutes.

10. Meanwhile, make the toppings. Toast the coconut by spreading it out in a thin layer on a baking sheet and baking in the 300°F oven 10-15 minutes, stirring every few minutes to help it toast evenly. Place all the chocolate in the top of a double boiler over simmering water and stir until almost melted. Remove from the heat and stir until completely melted and smooth.

11. To assemble cookies, place a small spoonful of caramel on top of each cookie. Top with a sprinkle of toasted coconut. Let cool.

12. Dip the bottom of each cookie in chocolate. Place on a parchment-lined baking sheet to set. Then drizzle the tops with chocolate. Let cookies sit about 1 hour for the chocolate to fully set up.

13. Enjoy! Store in an airtight container up to 5 days, or in the freezer up to 3 months.

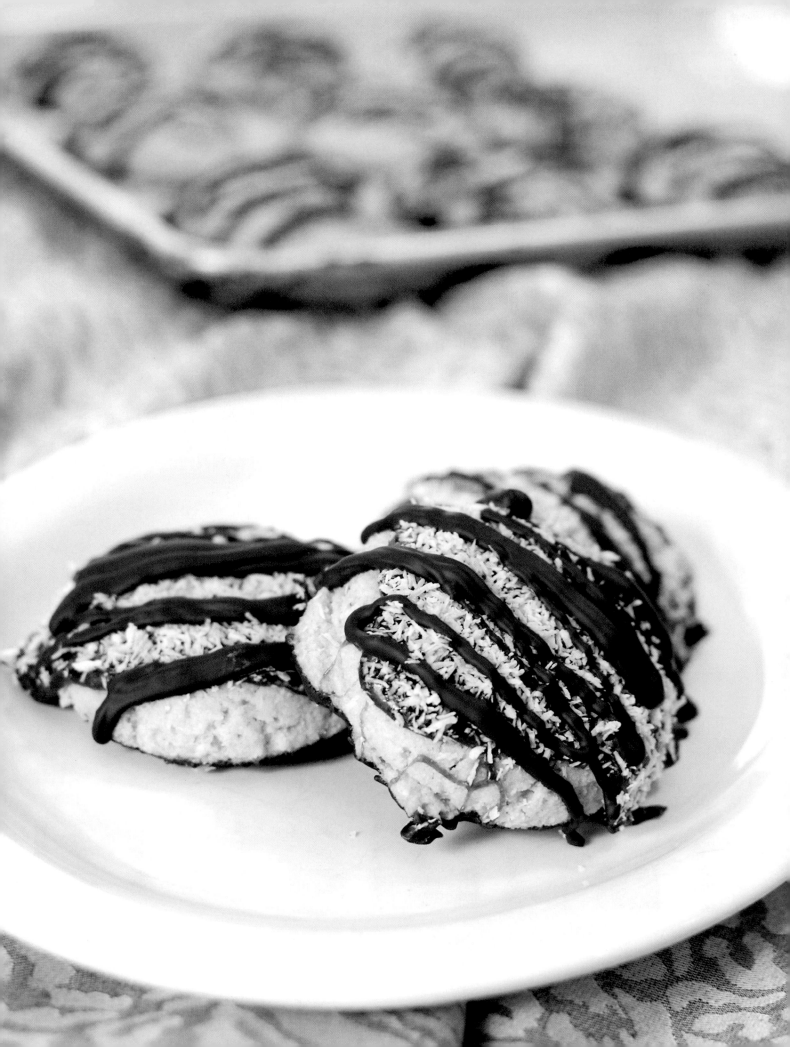

No-Bake Macadamia Thumbprints

with Whipped Chocolate Ganache

Makes 9 cookies
Dairy Free • Egg Free • Fish Free

Cookie

1 cup (150 g) roasted, salted macadamias

1 cup (90 g) unsweetened, finely shredded coconut

1 tsp pure vanilla extract

¼ cup (60 mL) coconut oil, melted

½ tsp orange zest (optional)

1 TBSP pure maple syrup

Whipped Ganache

3 TBSP coconut oil, melted

2 TBSP pure maple syrup

1 TBSP unsweetened cocoa powder

2 TBSP palm shortening

2 tsp arrowroot starch

We love a good no-bake cookie around our house because that means the kids can do most of the work. Hey, it's a good learning experience! Plus, the creamy macadamias and hint of sweet chocolaty goodness in the filling really hit the spot. We like ours with a touch of orange zest for another layer of flavor, but feel free to leave it out.

1. Make the cookies. Place the macadamias in a food processor and pulse into a coarse meal. Don't process too long or you'll end up with butter.

2. Add the remaining cookie ingredients and pulse until combined, about 30 seconds.

3. Scoop rounded tablespoons of dough and place on waxed-paper-lined baking sheets. Press your thumb into each ball to create a well. If cookies are too soft to hold their shape, place tray in the fridge for about 15 minutes or until cookies firm up enough to make the well in the center.

4. Meanwhile, make the ganache. Combine all the ganache ingredients in a small bowl and whip with a hand mixer until smooth and fluffy. Store in the fridge if not using right away; soften at room temperature before using.

5. Fill each cookie with ganache.

6. Refrigerate about an hour, until very firm. Enjoy! Store in an airtight container in the fridge up to 2 weeks, or in the freezer up to 3 months.

Note:
Your favorite sugar-free jam or jelly would make a great thumbprint fill-in as well!

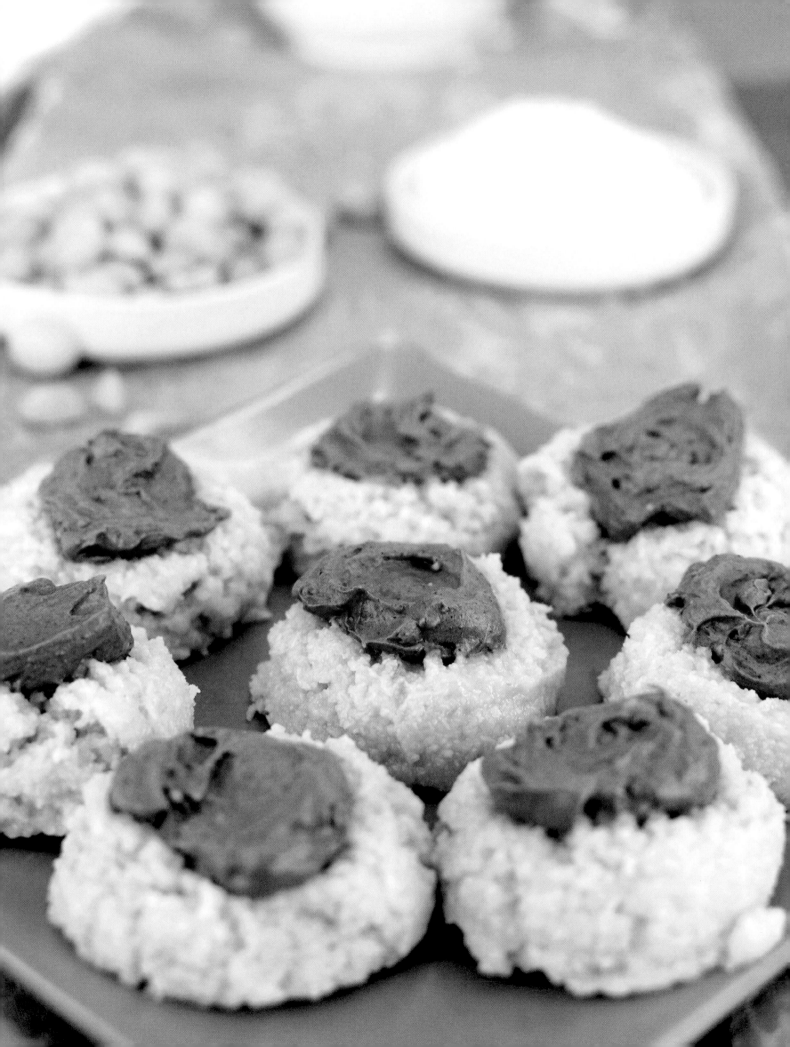

Pecan Sandies

Makes 9 cookies
Dairy Free • Fish Free

Dry Ingredients

1¾ cups (225 g) raw pecans

3 TBSP coconut flour, sifted

2 TBSP arrowroot starch

½ tsp baking soda

⅛ tsp sea salt

Wet Ingredients

1 egg

½ tsp pure vanilla extract

¼ cup (80 mL) pure maple syrup

2 TBSP coconut oil, melted

Add In

⅓ cup (50 g) raw chopped pecans

Pecans with maple syrup—what's not to love? Besides, pecans are higher in omega-3 fatty acids than almonds and have about half as much omega-6 as walnuts, which make them a nice baking alternative. So don't get into a rut thinking almond flour is your only choice for Paleo baking; experiment by making a few of your own nut flours for variety in both nutrients and flavor.

1. Place the pecans in a food processor and pulse into a coarse meal.

2. Place the ground pecans and the remaining dry ingredients in a medium bowl and stir to combine.

3. Add the wet ingredients to the dry and combine with a hand mixer until well blended.

4. Stir in the chopped pecans.

5. Place the dough on plastic wrap, roll into a 2-inch diameter log, and refrigerate overnight, or freeze 1-2 hours or until very firm.

6. Preheat the oven to 350°F.

7. Slice log into ¼-inch rounds. Place rounds on a parchment-lined baking sheet.

8. Bake about 11-13 minutes, or until browned on the edges.

9. Cool on trays for 5 minutes, then transfer to wire racks to cool completely. Store in an airtight container up to 4 days, or in the freezer up to 3 months.

Note:
To make softer cookies, you can scoop and bake immediately, but don't forget to preheat the oven when you start!

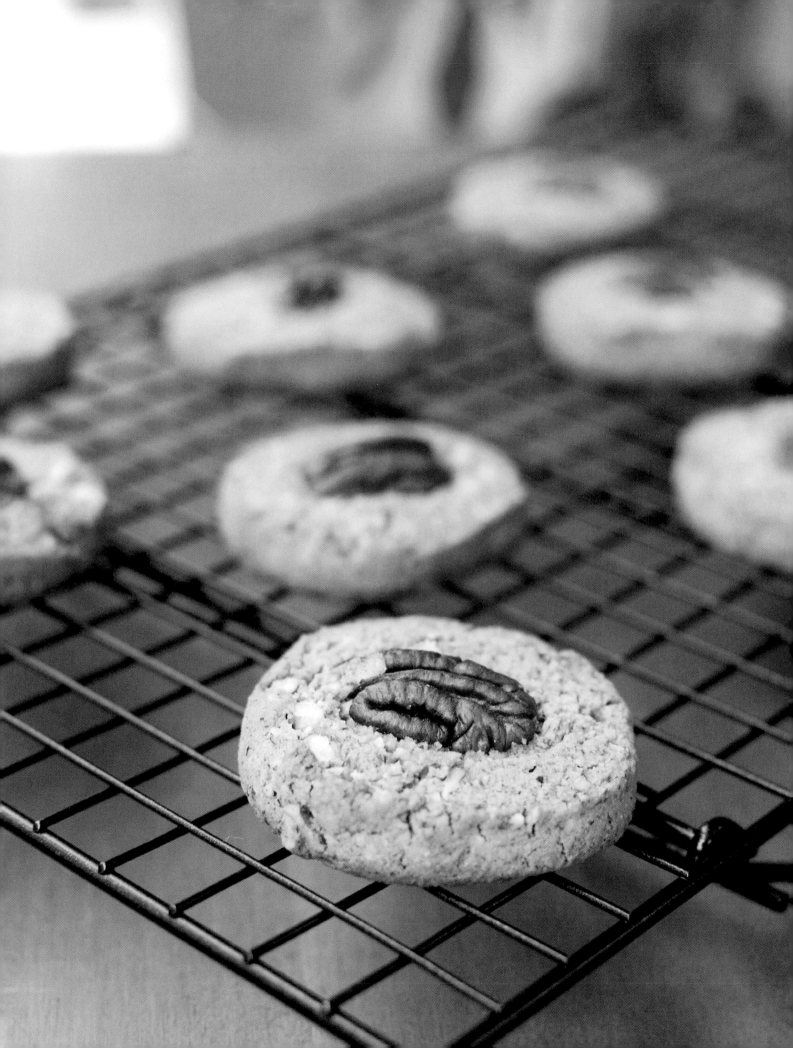

Graham Crackers

Makes 24 Graham Crackers
Dairy Free • Nut Free • Fish Free

Dry Ingredients

¼ cup (25 g) coconut flour, sifted

¼ cup (30 g) tapioca starch

¼ cup (30 g) arrowroot starch

1 tsp baking powder

½ tsp baking soda

1½ tsp cinnamon

Wet Ingredients

⅓ cup (80 mL) pure maple syrup

1 egg

2 tsp pure vanilla extract

¼ cup (60 mL) coconut oil, melted

Yes, this recipe is for graham crackers. Yes, they are crunchy and taste like graham crackers. No, they do not crumble in your hands, and no, they do not taste like a pile of almonds. Really! As a matter of fact, this recipe doesn't even use almond flour, believe it or not. I know! It's a lot to take in. But there's more! These crunchy little crackers also store beautifully for up to a week in an airtight container, so you can make them ahead of time for camping trips or picnics. Bring on summer!

1. Preheat oven to 350°F.

2. Place the dry ingredients in a medium bowl and whisk to combine.

3. Add the maple syrup, egg and vanilla extract. Mix well with a hand mixer.

4. With the mixer on low, slowly add the coconut oil. Blend well to incorporate. Let the dough rest for 3 minutes.

5. Pat the dough into a disc, cover in plastic wrap and refrigerate 15 minutes.

6. Place refrigerated dough between 2 pieces parchment paper (big enough to fit on your baking sheet) and roll to a ¼-inch thick rectangle. Remove top piece of parchment, place bottom piece with the dough on the baking sheet.

7. Using a sharp knife, score the dough lengthwise into 6 sections, then across into 4 sections. Or you can make any size crackers by scoring however you'd like. You don't have to conform here.

8. Poke dough all over with fork.

9. Bake 8 minutes, then pull the tray out and carefully (use a spatula) separate the crackers. Return the crackers to the oven and bake 5-8 minutes more, or until centers are cooked and edges are golden.

10. Cool on trays on wire racks. Store in an airtight container up to 5 days or freeze for up to 3 months.

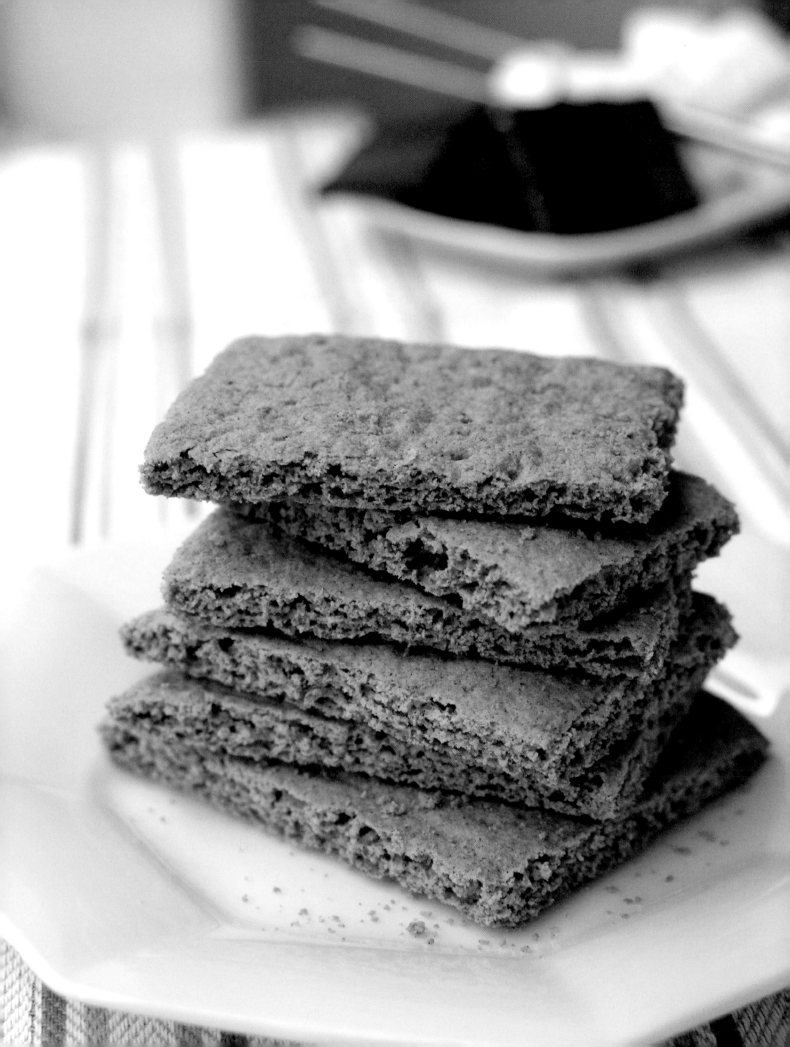

Decadent Brownies

Makes 16 brownies

Dairy Free • Fish Free • Nut Free

Step 1

2 oz (56 g) dark chocolate, chopped

3 TBSP full-fat coconut milk

¼ cup (25 g) unsweetened cocoa powder

3 TBSP coconut oil, melted

Step 2

3 TBSP arrowroot starch

¼ cup (25 g) coconut flour, sifted

¼ tsp baking soda

Pinch sea salt

Step 3

½ cup (120 mL) pure maple syrup

¼ cup (60 mL) olive oil

2 eggs, whisked

¼ cup (60 g) canned pumpkin

These chocolaty cake-like bites of heaven will not let you down when you're craving that classic brownie flavor and slightly crackly top! I didn't want the nutty flavor and texture that comes with almond flour to mess with my ideal brownie, so I gave up a little fudginess to maximize the traditional flavor I was after. I think it was worth it!

1. Preheat the oven to 350°F.

2. Place all the Step 1 ingredients in a small saucepan over low heat until melted. Remove from heat.

3. Place all the Step 2 ingredients in a medium bowl and whisk to combine.

4. Add the Step 1 chocolate mixture and all the Step 3 wet ingredients to the Step 2 dry ingredients. Blend well with a hand mixer.

5. Pour the batter into a greased 8-by-8-inch glass baking dish. Bake 25 minutes, or until a toothpick inserted in the center comes out clean.

6. Cool completely on a wire rack. Cut brownies into squares and enjoy! Store leftovers in an airtight container up to 2 days (brownies will get softer and more cake-like the next day) or freeze up to 3 months.

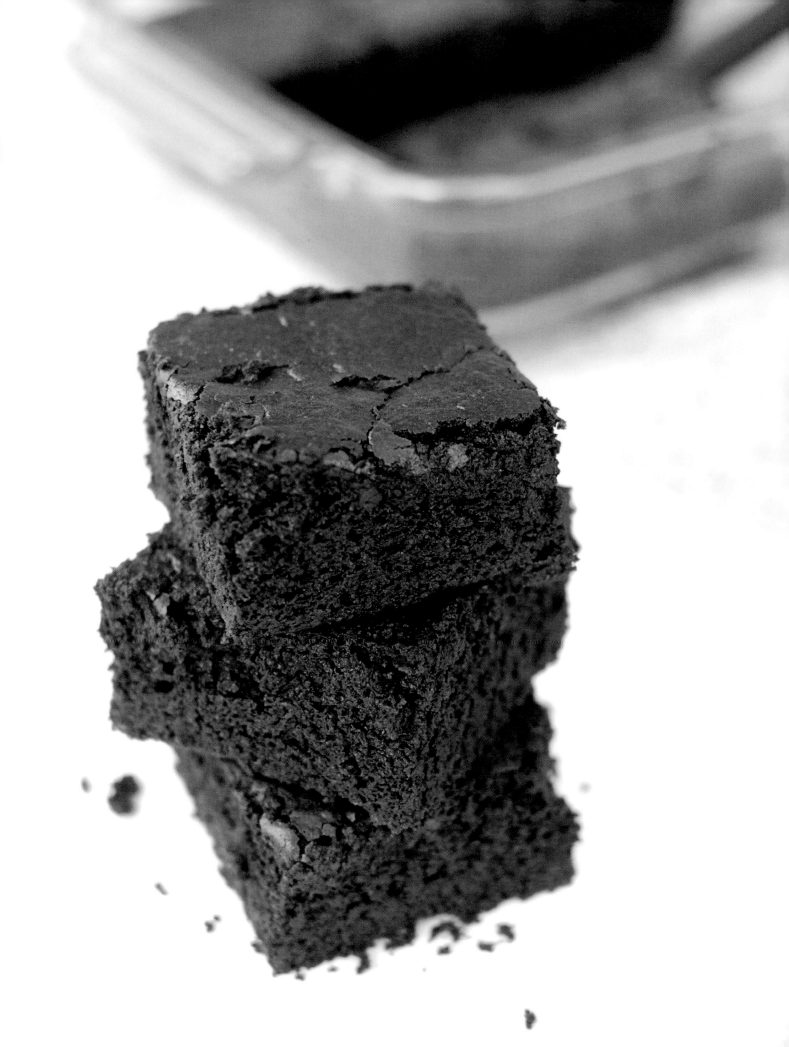

Vanilla Brownie Cheesecake

Fish Free • Nut Free

Crust

2½ cups (350 g) Brownie Crumbs (page 88)

¼ cup (60 mL) coconut oil, melted

Filling

16 oz (450 g) cream cheese, softened

½ cup (115 g) sour cream, room temperature

½ cup (120 g) mascarpone cheese, softened

1 cup (240 mL) pure maple syrup

2 tsp pure vanilla extract

1 vanilla bean, split and scraped

1 TBSP arrowroot starch

6 large eggs, room temperature

Topping

1 cup (230 g) sour cream

½ tsp pure vanilla extract

1 TBSP pure maple syrup

I know some Paleo enthusiasts will cringe at this dairy-loaded dessert, but for those who occasionally partake in dairy from grass-fed animals, this creamy traditional dessert can save you from jumping headfirst into some feedlot-dairy cheesecake at the bakery. This is my birthday cake of choice, so I simply choose high-quality products, enjoy each and every bite, and then I'm done until my next special day. Remember to select dairy from pastured cows, local if possible, and full-fat versions. Plan to make this a day before you need it so it has time to set up properly.

1. Preheat the oven to 350°F.

2. Grease a 9-inch springform pan. Place it on a baking sheet.

3. Place the crust ingredients in a small bowl and mix. Press the crust into the springform pan, smoothing it across the bottom and about three-quarters of the way up the sides.

4. Bake 8-10 minutes. Place tray on a wire rack to cool.

5. Turn the oven up to 450°F.

6. Make the filling. Cut the cream cheese into chunks and place in the bowl of an electric mixer, fit with the paddle attachment. Mix on medium speed for 3 minutes until smooth. Add the sour cream and mascarpone cheese. Mix for another 2 minutes, until combined and smooth. Add the maple syrup, vanilla, vanilla bean scrapings, and arrowroot starch. Mix until combined. Add the eggs, one at a time, beating after each until fully incorporated. Scrape down the sides as you go.

7. With the pan still on the baking sheet, pour the filling into the cooled crust.

8. Bake for 15 minutes.

9. Turn the oven down to 250°F and bake for 60 minutes more.

10. Meanwhile, make the topping. Place all the topping ingredients in a small bowl and stir with a spoon to combine.

11. Remove the cake from the oven (after the 60 minutes) and spread the topping over it. Return it to the oven.

12. Turn the oven off, open the door a crack, and leave the cake in the oven for 30 minutes more.

13. Remove from the oven and carefully run a knife around the edge of the pan to loosen the cake from the sides.

14. Let cool completely on a wire rack before covering with plastic wrap. Refrigerate overnight.

15. Remove side ring from the springform pan, slice the cake, and serve! Store in an airtight container in the fridge up to 3 days, or in the freezer up to 2 months.

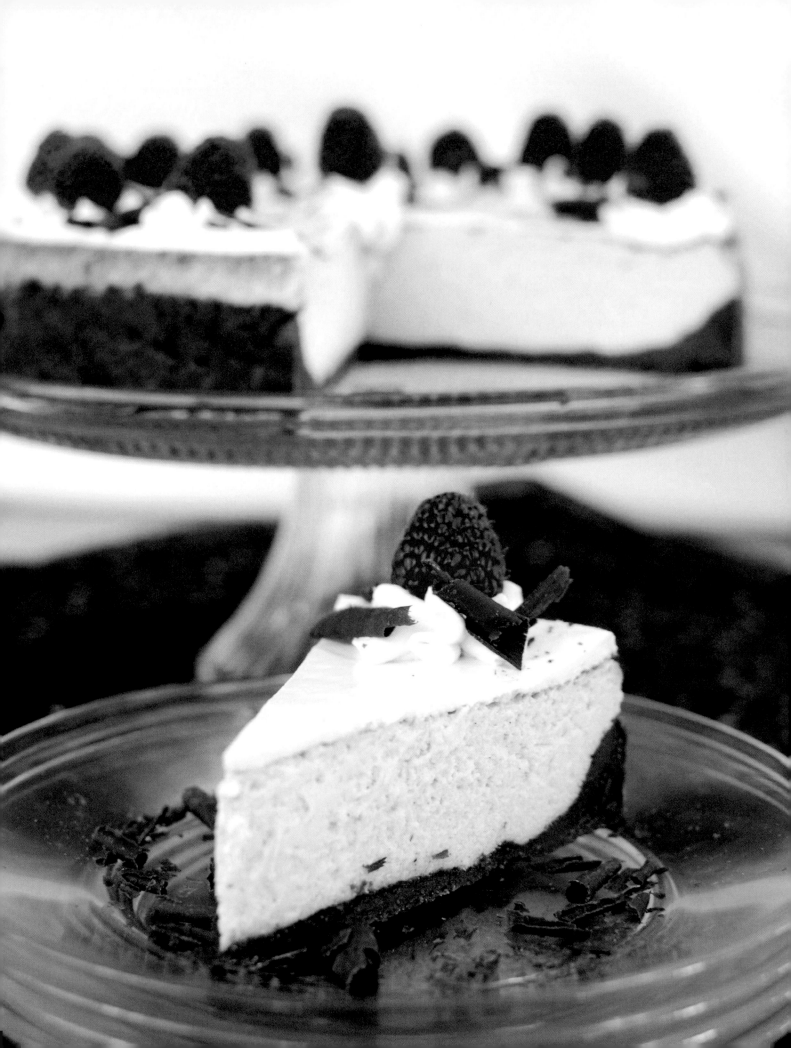

Egg White Bread

Makes 8

Dairy Free* • Fish Free • Nut Free

3 eggs, separated

3 TBSP canned coconut milk (full-fat or light)

1 TBSP coconut flour, sifted

1 tsp very soft ghee (or coconut oil*, melted)

1 tsp pure maple syrup or raw honey

¼ tsp cream of tartar

Pinch sea salt

This "bread" came about totally by accident. For me, this is no surprise. A lot of my cooking is accidental. Anyway, I was trying for a macaroon-type cookie base, but the result was more like a bread with a buttery flavor, and my family fell in love with it. We like this as a side dish every so often, or as a hamburger bun when the mood strikes. The texture is eggy, but the flavor is buttery. Hard to explain really. You'll just have to make them to know what I mean!

1. Preheat the oven to 300°F.

2. Place the egg yolks, coconut milk, coconut flour, ghee, and maple syrup in a small bowl and mix with a hand mixer until well combined.

3. Place the egg whites, cream of tartar, and sea salt in a separate bowl and beat with a hand mixer (with clean beaters) on high until fluffy and peaks form.

4. Gently fold the egg white mixture into the egg yolk mixture just until blended. Do not overmix. You want to keep as much fluffiness as possible.

5. Use an ice-cream size scoop and place 8 mounds of dough onto parchment-lined baking sheets.

6. Bake 20 minutes, or until they are a nice golden brown.

7. Enjoy warm, or let them cool to use as a sandwich bread or hamburger bun.

8. Leftovers tend to dry out quickly, so I recommend freezing them in an airtight container, and be sure to separate them with waxed paper so they don't stick together.

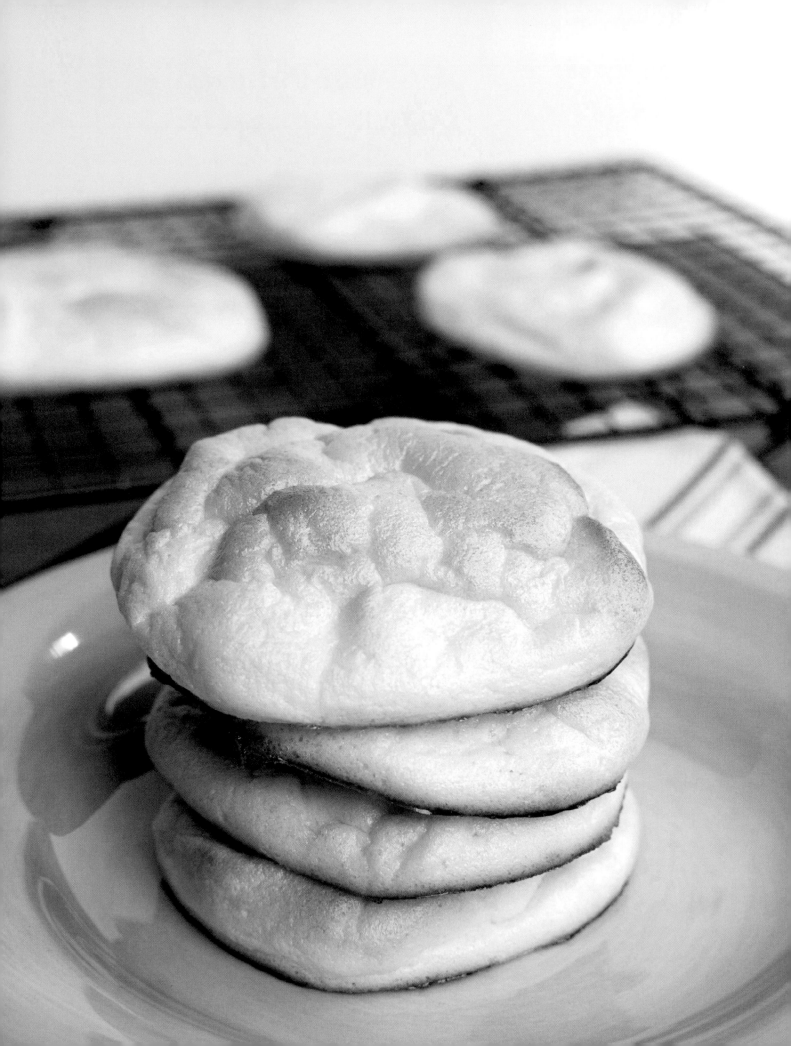

Sweet Potato Thyme Biscuits

Makes 6 biscuits
Dairy Free • Fish Free

A fantastic addition to the Thanksgiving table, these mouthwatering biscuits will soon be part of your family traditions. Crispy on the edges and soft in the middle means they disappear quickly, so make plenty! And why not make things easy on yourself by making a double batch and freezing before the big day? Just heat and eat. Now that's something to be thankful for.

Dry Ingredients

¾ cup (90 g) almond flour

2 TBSP coconut flour, sifted

¼ tsp sea salt

1 tsp baking powder

Wet Ingredients

½ cup (120 g) cooked, mashed sweet potato

2 TBSP coconut milk (full-fat or light)

2 TBSP raw honey

3 eggs

¼ cup (60 mL) coconut oil, melted

Add In

1 tsp chopped fresh thyme

1. Preheat the oven to 350°F.

2. Place the dry ingredients in a medium bowl and whisk to combine.

3. Add the wet ingredients, except the coconut oil, to the dry ingredients and stir with a spoon to combine.

4. Add the coconut oil and thyme and stir until combined.

5. Let the batter sit 5 minutes to thicken.

6. Use an ice-cream size scoop and place 6 mounds of dough onto a parchment-lined baking sheet. Bake 25-30 minutes, or until browned and firm to the touch.

7. Place baking sheet on a wire rack until biscuits are cool. Store in an airtight container up to 2 days, or freeze up to 3 months. To serve from frozen, simply thaw at room temperature, cover with foil and bake in a 350°F oven until heated through.

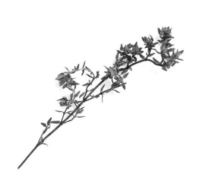

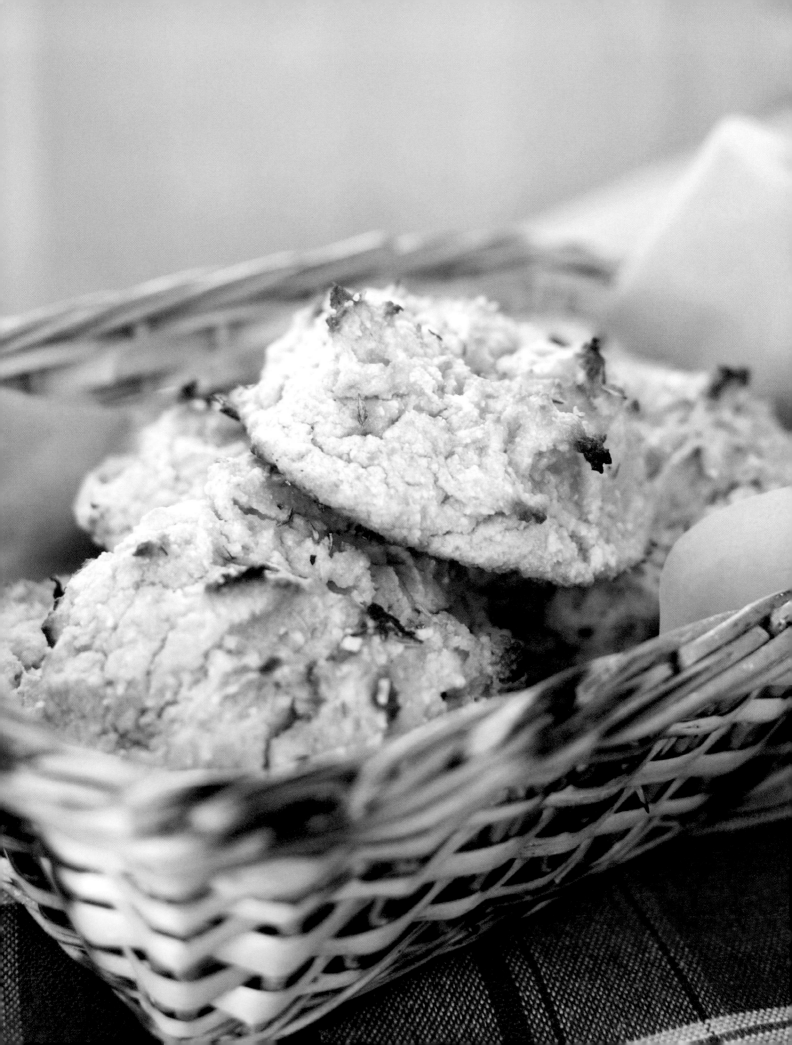

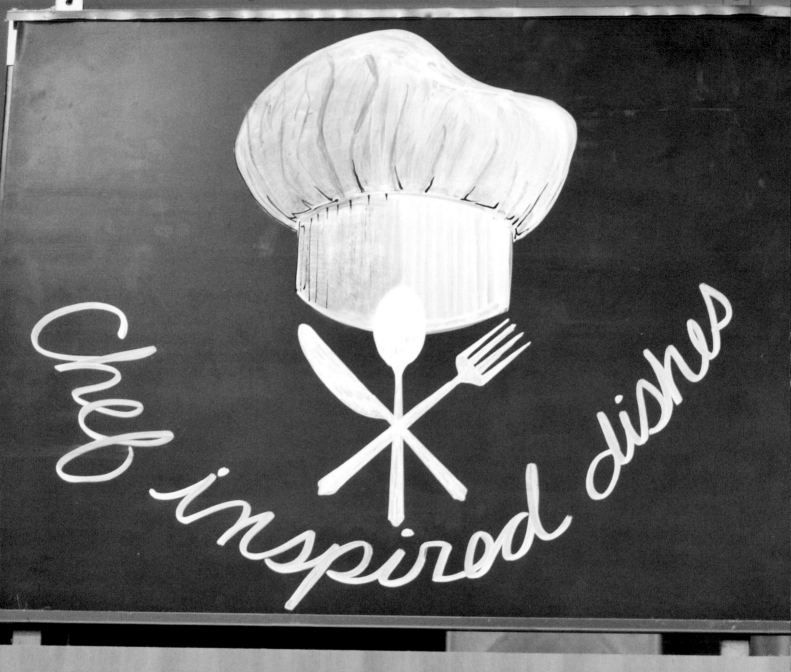

Chef inspired dishes

Our Prepared Fare

Today's Specials

Tropical Macadamia Bars

Makes about 20 bars

Dairy Free • Egg Free • Fish Free

½ cup (75 g) chopped unsulfured, unsweetened dried mango

1 cup (150 g) roasted, salted macadamia nuts

1 tsp minced fresh ginger

2 TBSP sesame seeds

⅓ cup (30 g) unsweetened finely shredded coconut

2 TBSP raw honey

These dense little bars pack a wallop of flavor and nutrition. Not to mention that they are super simple to make. Perfect for school lunchboxes or snacks on the road, these nutty, gingery treats are meant to be enjoyed anywhere!

1. If needed, place the mango in a bowl with hot water for 15 minutes to soften.

2. Place the remaining ingredients in a food processor and pulse until nuts are ground semi-fine but still slightly chunky.

3. Place the mixture in a plastic-wrap-lined 8-by-8-inch pan.

4. Drain the mangoes and add to the macadamia mixture, mixing them in by hand to evenly distribute.

5. Place a piece of plastic wrap or parchment paper on top of the mixture to prevent sticking and press down firmly to compress the mixture as much as you can to ensure that it sticks together.

6. Refrigerate until firm, about 3 hours. To hurry things along, you can place in the freezer for an hour or two.

7. Cut into small bars or squares. Store in an airtight container in the fridge up to 5 days, or in the freezer up to 3 months.

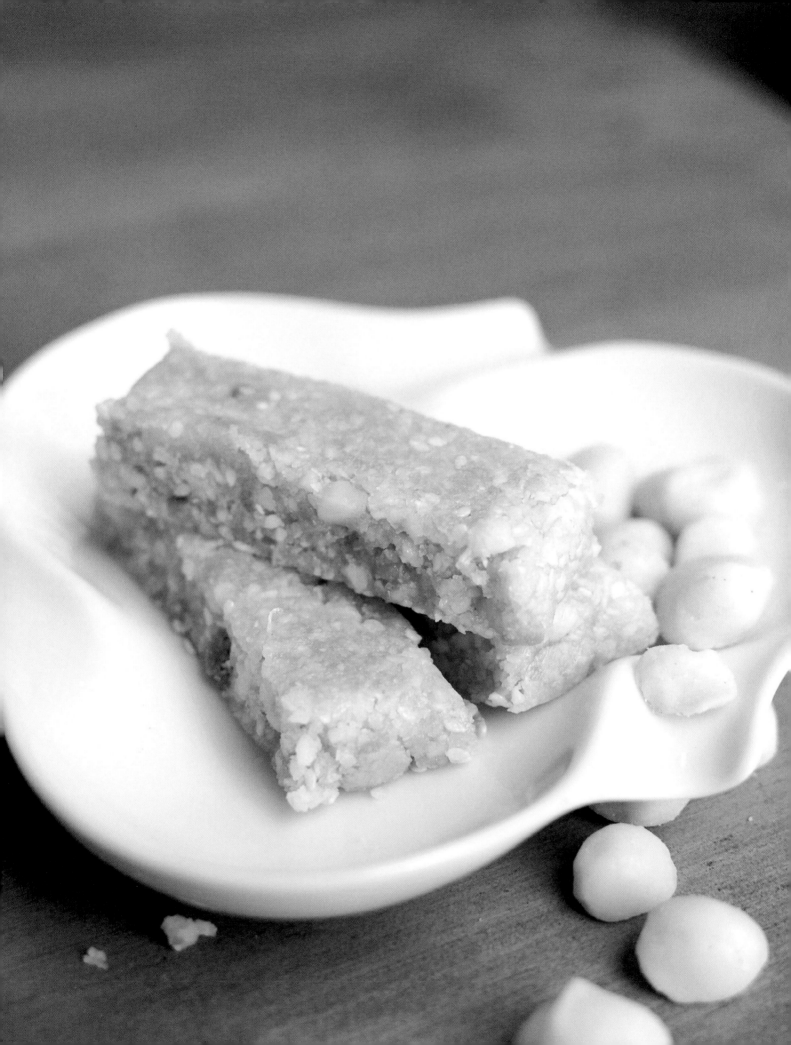

Granola Bars

Makes 16 bars
Dairy Free • Egg Free • Fish Free

Wet Ingredients

¼ cup (60 mL) coconut oil

¼ cup (60 mL) pure maple syrup

¼ cup (60 g) unsweetened almond butter

Dry Ingredients

⅓ cup (50 g) raw pumpkin seeds

½ cup (75 g) roasted, salted sunflower seeds

⅓ cup (50 g) roasted, salted almond slivers

¼ cup (40 g) mini chocolate chips (Enjoy Life brand)

⅓ cup (50 g) raisins

Here's my Paleo twist on a traditional granola bar! Puréed nuts and seeds formed into bars are great for an occasional snack, but because they are ground into tiny pieces, it's very easy to over-indulge. I really like that this recipe uses whole nuts and seeds, making it easier not to over-do it.

1. Preheat the oven to 325°F. Line an 8-by-8-inch pan with parchment paper and grease with coconut oil.

2. Place the wet ingredients in a small saucepan over low heat, stirring occasionally just until melted and combined. Set aside to cool, about 15 minutes.

3. Place the dry ingredients in a medium bowl. Pour the melted wet ingredients over the dry ingredients and stir to combine.

4. Spoon into the prepared pan. Place a sheet of waxed paper on top and press down firmly to flatten.

5. Bake 25-30 minutes, or until bubbly and golden.

6. Remove from the oven and let cool for 15 minutes. Cut into bars.

7. Cool completely. Place bars in an airtight container in the refrigerator to fully firm up.

8. Store in an airtight container in the fridge up to a week, or in the freezer up to 3 months.

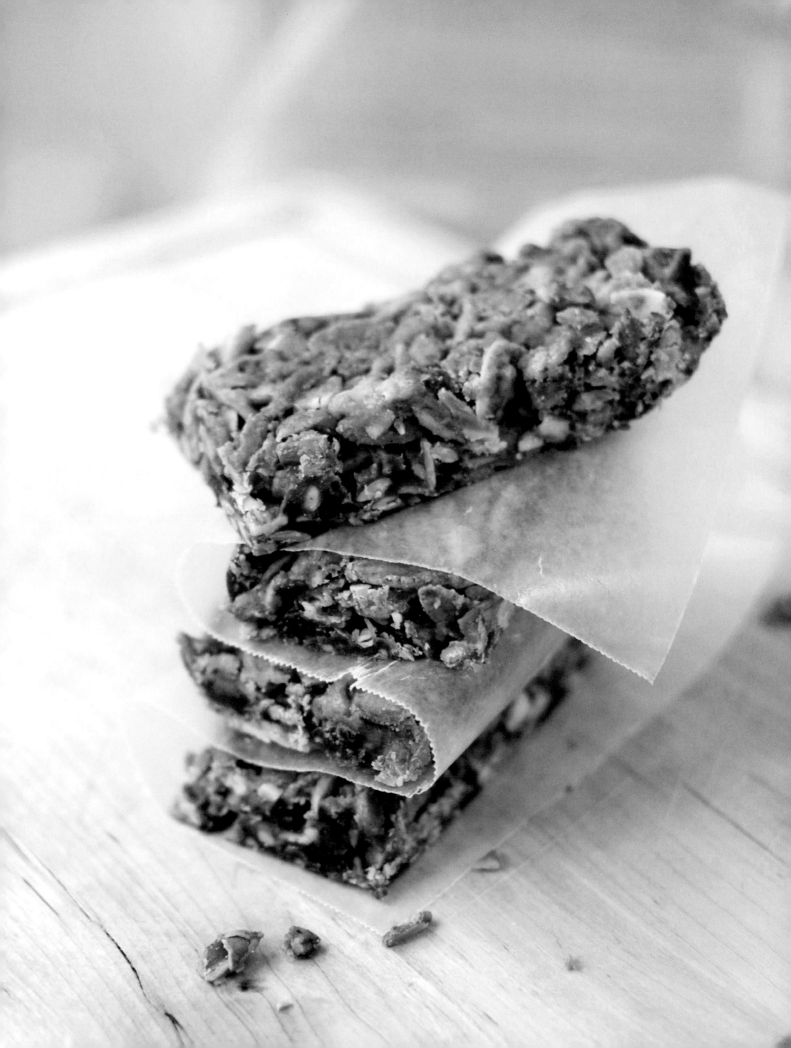

Fruit Dip

Makes about 1 ½ cups
Dairy Free • Egg Free • Fish Free • Nut Free

1 (1.2 oz) package unsweetened, unsulfured freeze-dried strawberries (30 g, about 1¼ cups)

⅓ cup (80 mL) coconut oil, melted

¼ cup (48 g) palm shortening

3 TBSP coconut nectar, pure maple syrup, or raw honey

½ tsp pure vanilla extract

¼ cup (60 g) coconut butter, softened

Pinch sea salt

Back in college, when I knew everything, I never worried about what I ate. Which is why I came to adore a ridiculously luscious, stupidly sugary strawberry fruit dip made with powdered sugar, "whipped topping," and marshmallow cream. Now I get a headache just thinking about it! Strawberries are so sweet on their own, who needed a one-pound bag of powdered sugar to "accent" the flavor? So much for knowing everything back then. Nowadays when my kiddos beg for something fun in their lunches, I make this gorgeous dip, which really does highlight the strawberry flavor, without burying it in sugar.

1. Place the strawberries in a food processor and process until they turn into powder.

2. Add the remaining ingredients and pulse until fully combined.

3. Place mixture in a covered bowl and refrigerate until semi-firm, about 1 hour.

4. Blend again in the food processor or with a hand mixer to fluff it up.

5. Serve with fruit for dipping!

Note:
Use freeze-dried bananas, raspberries, or blueberries for other fun dip flavors.

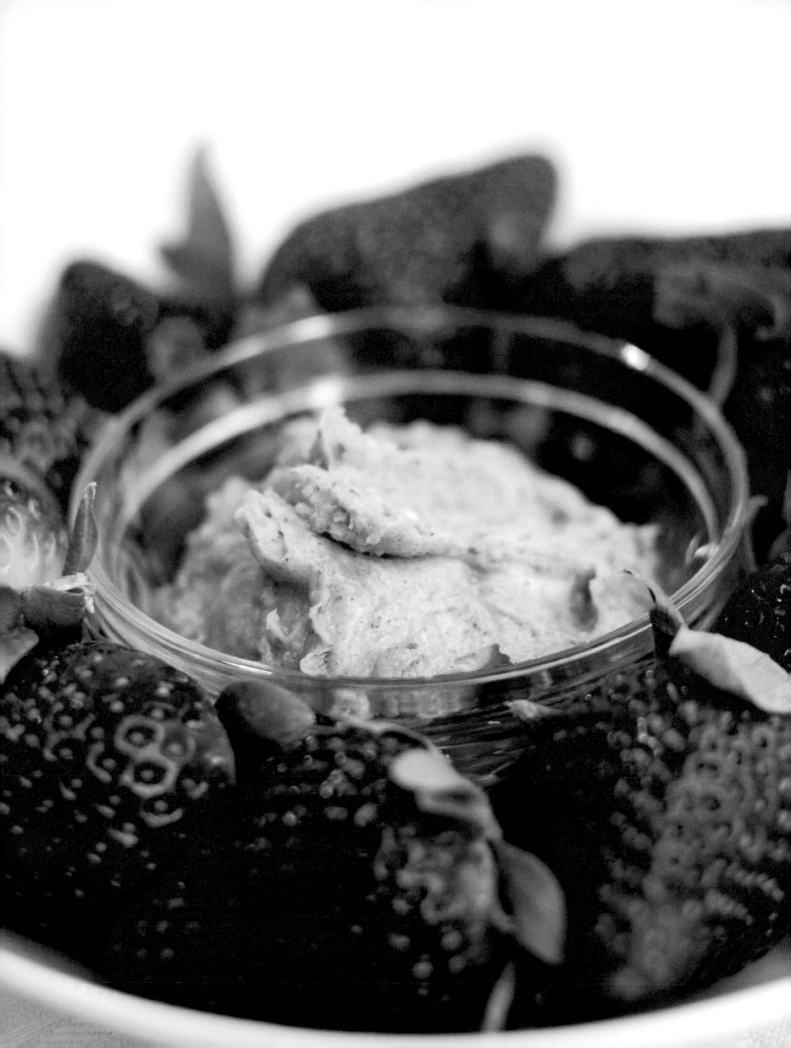

Fruit Jerky

Makes 12 strips

Dairy Free • Egg Free • Fish Free • Nut Free

3 cups (450 g) fresh or thawed frozen fruit (pitted cherries, strawberries, blueberries, raspberries, mango, pineapple, etc.)

My kiddos love making our own healthy version of fruit leather because they get to control everything—choosing the fruit to use, pushing the buttons on the food processor, pouring the purée into the pan, and then checking on its progress about 100 zillion times until it's ready! But it's worth the wait when you bite into the tart, concentrated flavor of the jerky knowing there's nothing else in there but fruit—no sugar, no thickeners, no artificial anything. And don't worry if you don't get the texture just right the first time. We over dried ours the first time we made this and ended up with fruit "chips." But they were still great, and the kids scarfed them up, so we're calling it a successful mistake!

1. Heat the oven to its lowest setting, about 150°F to 170°F.

2. Place the fruit in a blender or food processor and purée until smooth. Strain seeds if desired.

3. Line a rimmed baking sheet with parchment paper and grease with coconut oil.

4. Spread the fruit purée evenly over parchment.

5. Place the baking sheet in the oven and leave the door open slightly so the oven doesn't get too warm. It will take 2-4 hours to dry out your fruit, depending on how thick the purée is.

6. Let the purée cool to room temperature, then slice into strips. Carefully peel strips off of the parchment paper. To store, roll fruit strips around pieces of waxed paper and place in an airtight container for up to a week.

Note:

If the edges of the jerky start drying out too much (after about 2 hours) simply brush them with water to keep them as moist as the center. If you don't, the edges will become fruit chips and the center fruit jerky—two recipes in one!

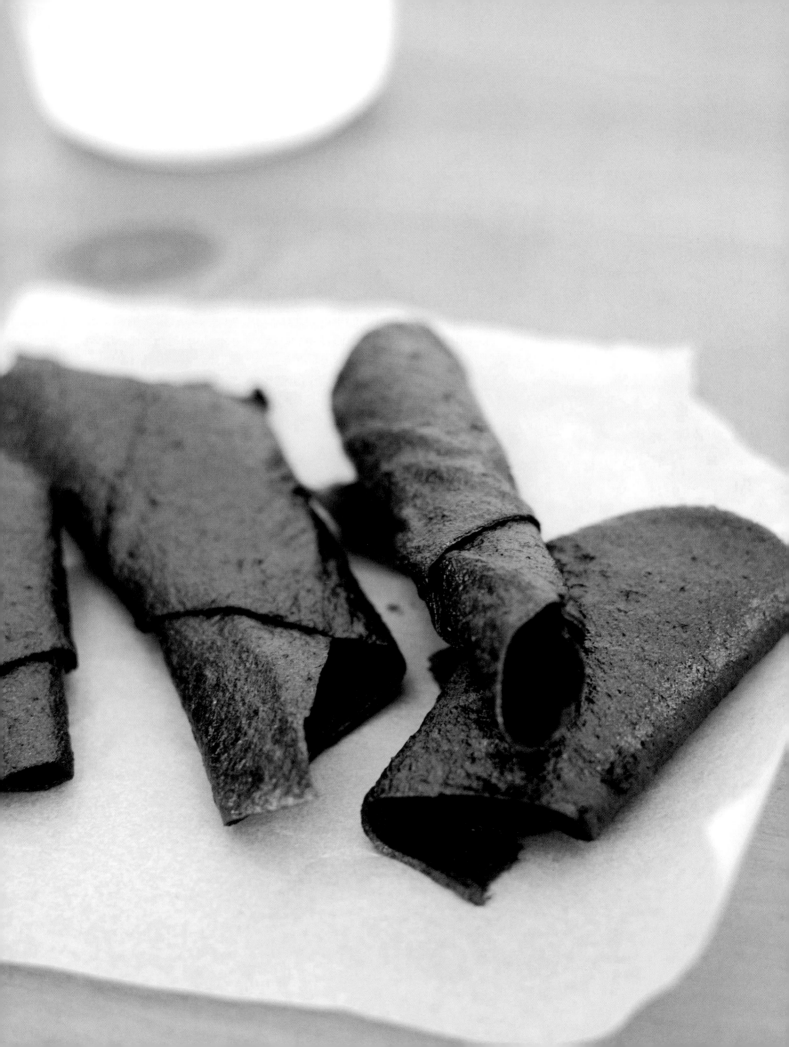

Italian Herb Crackers

Makes 30 crackers
Dairy Free • Fish Free

Dry Ingredients

½ cup (75 g) almond flour

¼ cup (25 g) coconut flour, sifted

¼ tsp sea salt

¼ tsp freshly ground black pepper

1 tsp Italian seasoning

Wet Ingredients

1 egg

1 TBSP coconut oil, melted

Once in a great while a little cracker comes in handy to pair with a tasty Onion Dip (page 126) during the big game or with some uncured ham and sliced veggies on a road trip. My family devoured these crunchy snacks, managing to say that they were "delicious and cheesy tasting" between bites, which is pretty remarkable considering that they are 100 percent cheese-free! Have fun and play with the seasonings to create your own favorite flavor combinations!

1. Preheat the oven to 350°F.

2. Place the dry ingredients in a medium bowl and whisk to combine.

3. Add the egg and mix well with a hand mixer.

4. With the mixer on low, slowly add the coconut oil. Blend well. Use your hands if you'd like!

5. Place the dough on a parchment-lined baking sheet and press into a rectangle ⅛-inch thick using your hands. Use a piece of waxed paper on top of the dough if it sticks to your hands. Try not to let the edges get too thin or they'll burn.

6. Using a sharp knife, score the dough lengthwise into 6 sections, then across into 5 sections.

7. Bake 6 minutes, then pull the tray out and carefully separate the crackers with a spatula. Return the crackers to the oven and bake 6-9 minutes more, or until centers are cooked and edges are golden.

8. Cool on the tray on wire racks. Store in an airtight container up to 5 days, or freeze up to a month.

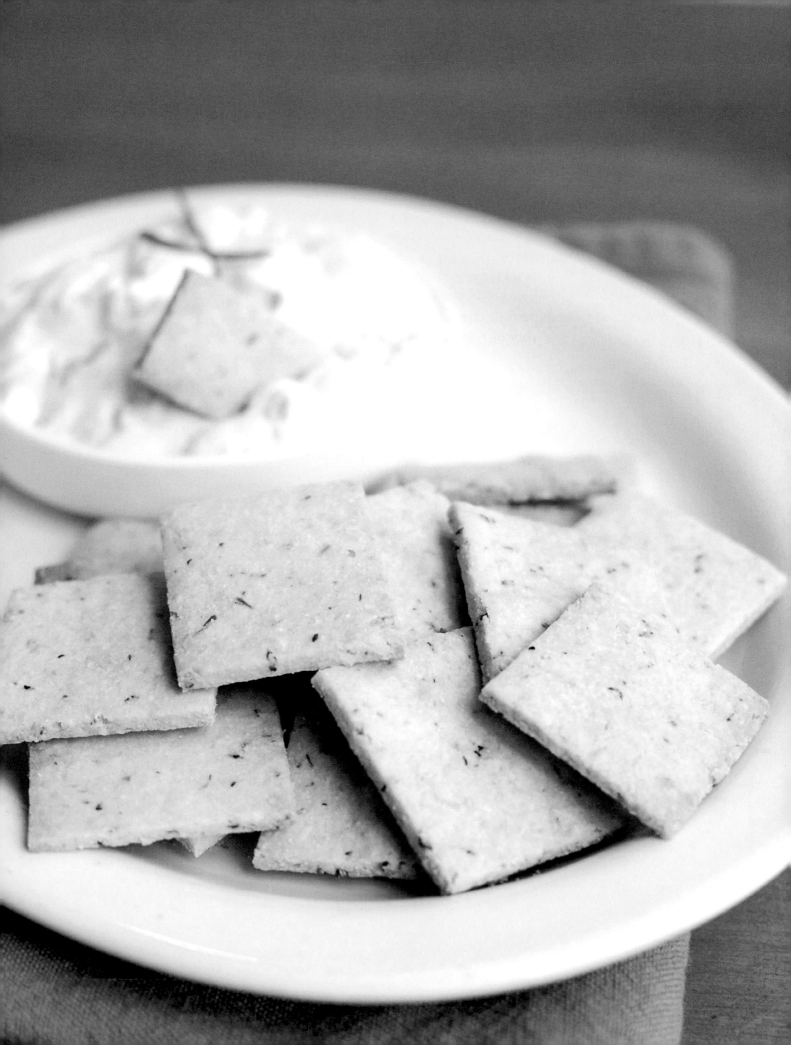

Seeded Crackers

Makes 30 crackers

Dairy Free • Fish Free • Nut Free

Dry Ingredients

½ cup (50 g) raw sunflower seeds

¼ cup (25 g) raw pumpkin seeds

¼ cup (25 g) coconut flour, sifted

¼ cup (40 g) sesame seeds

2 tsp poppy seeds

¼ tsp sea salt

¼ tsp freshly ground black pepper

Wet Ingredients

1 egg

1½ TBSP coconut oil, melted

For those with nut intolerances, here is a seeded cracker that is perfectly crunchy and ready for Bacon Guacamole (page 122)! The sky's the limit with flavor combinations, so feel free to get a little crazy with your spice inspiration. Try adding cumin and chili powder for a smoky cracker, or how about rosemary and garlic? You can even turn these into a sweet snack by adding some maple syrup or honey and sprinkle the tops with cinnamon!

1. Preheat the oven to 350°F.

2. Place the sunflower seeds and pumpkin seeds in a food processor and pulse into a fine meal.

3. Place the seed meal and the remaining dry ingredients in a medium bowl and stir to combine.

4. Add the egg and blend well with a hand mixer.

5. With the mixer on low, slowly add the coconut oil. Blend well.

6. Place the dough on a parchment-lined baking sheet and press into a rectangle ⅛-inch thick using your hands. Place a piece of waxed paper on top of the dough if it sticks to your hands. Try not to let the edges get too thin or they'll burn.

7. Using a sharp knife, score the dough lengthwise into 6 sections, then across into 5 sections.

8. Bake 6 minutes, then pull the tray out and carefully separate the crackers with a spatula. Return the crackers to the oven and bake 6-9 minutes more, or until centers are cooked and edges are golden.

9. Cool on the tray on wire racks. Store in an airtight container up to 5 days, or freeze up to 1 month.

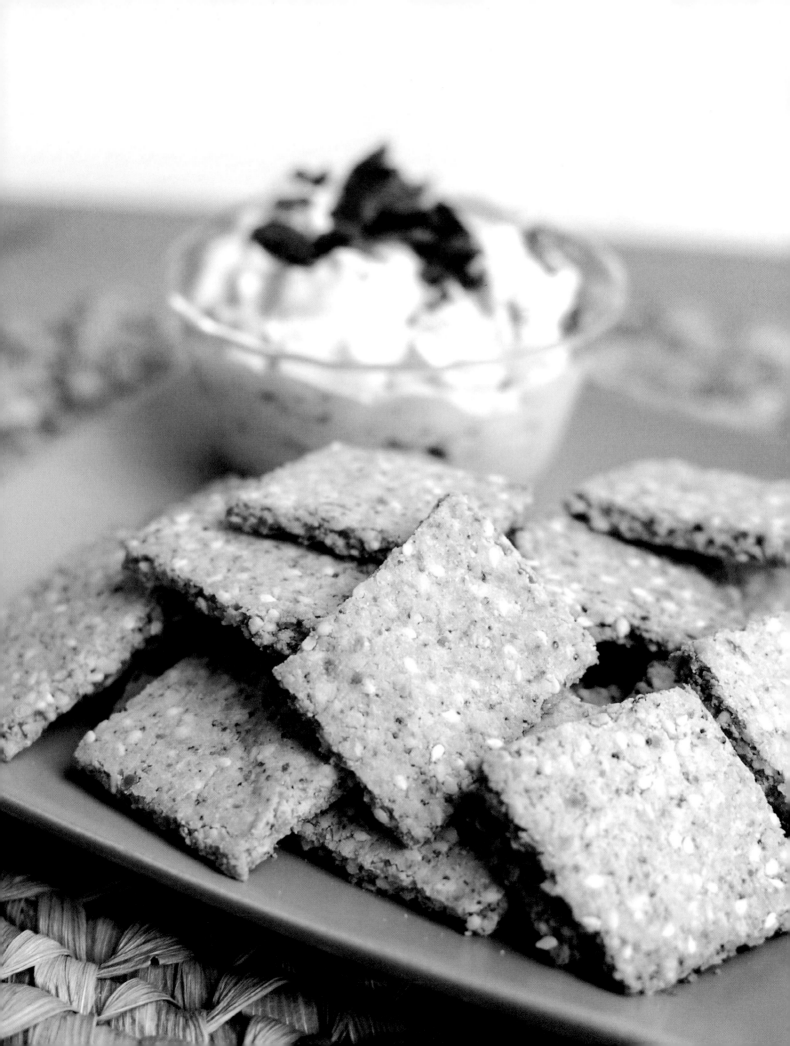

Bloody Mary Mix

Enough for a little troublemaking!
Dairy Free • Egg Free • Nut Free

1 46-oz (1.36-L) can tomato juice

1¾ cup (420 mL) beef broth (preferably homemade)

1-2 TBSP Worcestershire sauce (to taste)

Juice of 2 limes

½-1 tsp granulated garlic (to taste)

½-1 tsp celery salt (to taste)

½ tsp freshly ground black pepper (to taste)

1 tsp dill

3 or 4 shakes of your favorite hot sauce (to taste)

Sea salt (to taste)

Bacon-flavored vodka or plain vodka of your choice

Sometimes our family likes to have a leisurely brunch, and that's when this vivacious little cocktail gets to play a starring role. Yessssssss, alcohol is NOT meant for daily consumption, but once in a great while it's ok to splurge… responsibly. And while Robb Wolf's cocktail of choice entails tequila, memories of my college days has caused me to avoid that particular libation in favor of something a little less party-animal-ish. Sorry Robb! And, if sipping a Bloody Mary on Sunday morning wasn't decadent enough, try using bacon-flavored vodka and garnishing with bacon and celery. Yeah, I said bacon.

1. Place all the ingredients, except the vodka, in a large pitcher and mix until combined. Store in the fridge until ready to use. For best flavor, make 24 hours before needed.

2. To serve, pour 8 ounces mix into a glass with ice. Add 1 ounce of vodka.

3. Garnish with celery sticks and cooked bacon strips!

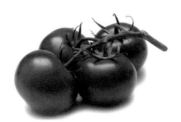

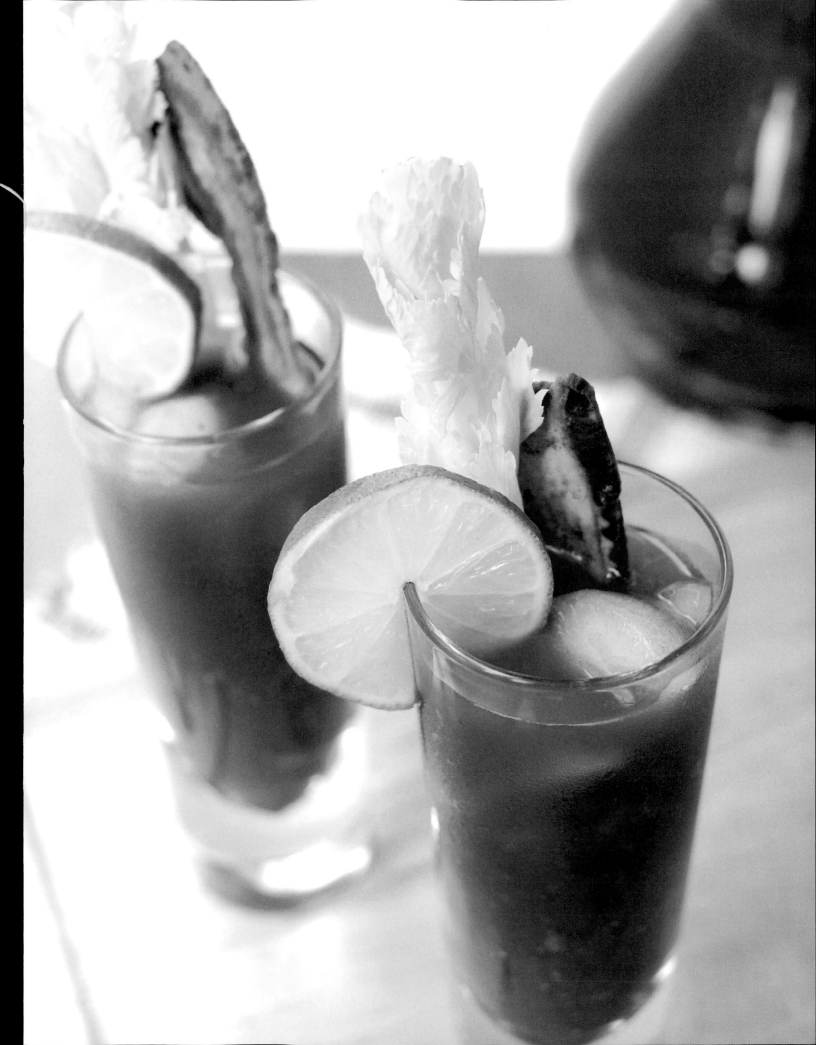

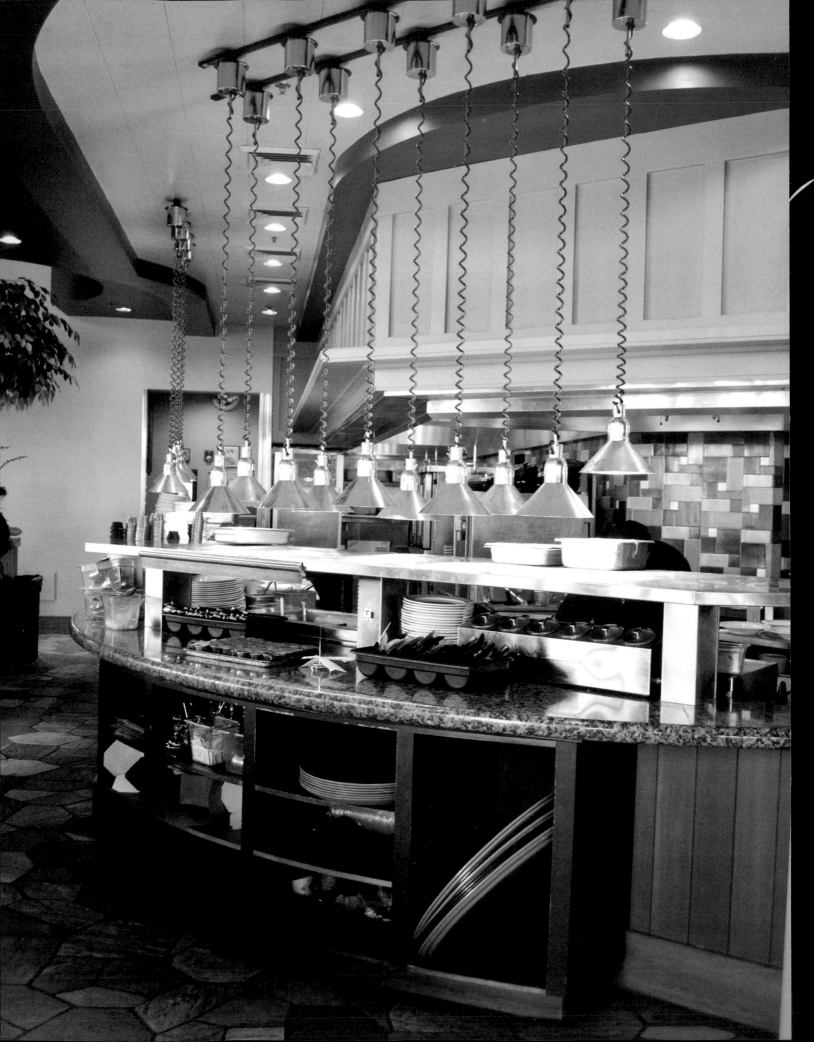

Restaurant Recreations

Breakfast Skillet

Makes 2 servings

Dairy Free • Fish Free • Nut Free

1 TBSP coconut oil, plus more if needed

1 cup (150 g) peeled and diced sweet potato (1 medium)

¼ cup (40 g) diced yellow onion

⅓ cup (50 g) diced red bell pepper

1 small pork chop or pork sirloin steak, cut into cubes (US Wellness Meats)

3 sausage links, diced (US Wellness Meats)

½ tsp marjoram

Pinch rosemary

Sea salt and freshly ground black pepper to taste

4 eggs

½ cup (75 g) chopped fresh spinach

Chopped fresh chives

½ avocado, sliced

There are a few national chains that offer breakfast skillets loaded with nitrate-filled feedlot meats, hormone-laden eggs, and chemical-infused non-organic white potatoes. Um, thanks, but I'll pass, and make my own version at home, using top-quality ingredients to create a morning meal that's sure not to be a health hazard. We love making these on lazy Sunday mornings in our Lodge cast iron skillets!

1. Heat 1 tablespoon oil in a 12-inch cast-iron skillet over medium heat. Add the sweet potato and cook until soft, about 8-10 minutes.

2. Add the onion and pepper and cook 3 minutes more.

3. Remove vegetables to a plate. Set aside.

4. Turn the heat to medium-high; add additional coconut oil to the pan if necessary. Add the pork chop and sausage. Season with marjoram, rosemary, salt, and pepper. Cook until browned and done, about 5 minutes. Remove to the plate with the vegetables.

5. Turn the heat to medium-low. Whisk the eggs and add to the pan. Scramble the eggs until almost cooked through. Add the spinach.

6. Add the vegetables and meat back to the pan and stir to combine.

7. When the eggs are cooked through, top with chives and avocado. Spoon onto two plates and serve!

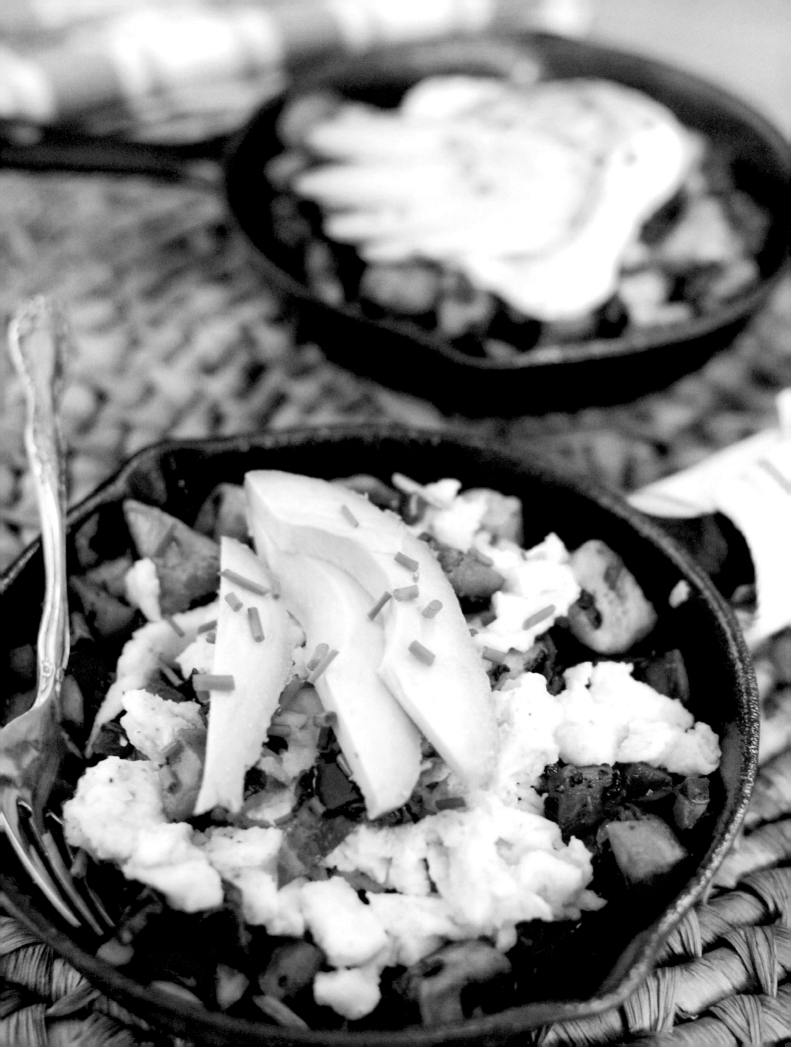

Breakfast Biscuit Bowls

Makes 4 bowls

Dairy Free • Fish Free

Biscuits

¾ cup (90 g) almond flour

⅓ cup (35 g) coconut flour, sifted

1 tsp baking soda

½ tsp sea salt

1 egg

3 TBSP coconut oil, melted

Filling

4 eggs, whisked

¼ cup (40 g) finely chopped chard, or spinach

½ cup (70 g) cooked ground beef or pork sausage (US Wellness Meats)

Sea salt and freshly ground black pepper to taste

Pinch granulated onion

Topping

Chopped fresh chives

For hectic mornings, this easy breakfast provides a tasty and filling meal, all packaged nicely in a biscuit to-go cup! But we enjoy the convenience even more when we're traveling because we can pack them in the cooler and heat them up in our hotel room microwave. No more jerky and trail mix breakfasts on the road!

1. Preheat the oven to 350°F.

2. Place the biscuit ingredients, except the coconut oil, in a medium bowl and use a hand mixer to combine. Add the coconut oil and mix well. Let sit 5 minutes to thicken, if necessary.

3. Divide the dough into 4 equal pieces and place each in a greased muffin cup, pressing down on the bottom and up the sides to form a cup.

4. Bake 10 minutes. Remove from the oven.

5. Place the filling ingredients in a medium bowl and whisk to combine. Divide among the baked biscuit cups.

6. Bake 12-15 minutes, or until egg is set.

7. Let the cups cool for a few minutes, then gently remove and serve! Top with chopped fresh chives, if desired.

Note:
These freeze well. Simply cool completely and freeze in airtight containers. To enjoy, thaw and reheat in the microwave.

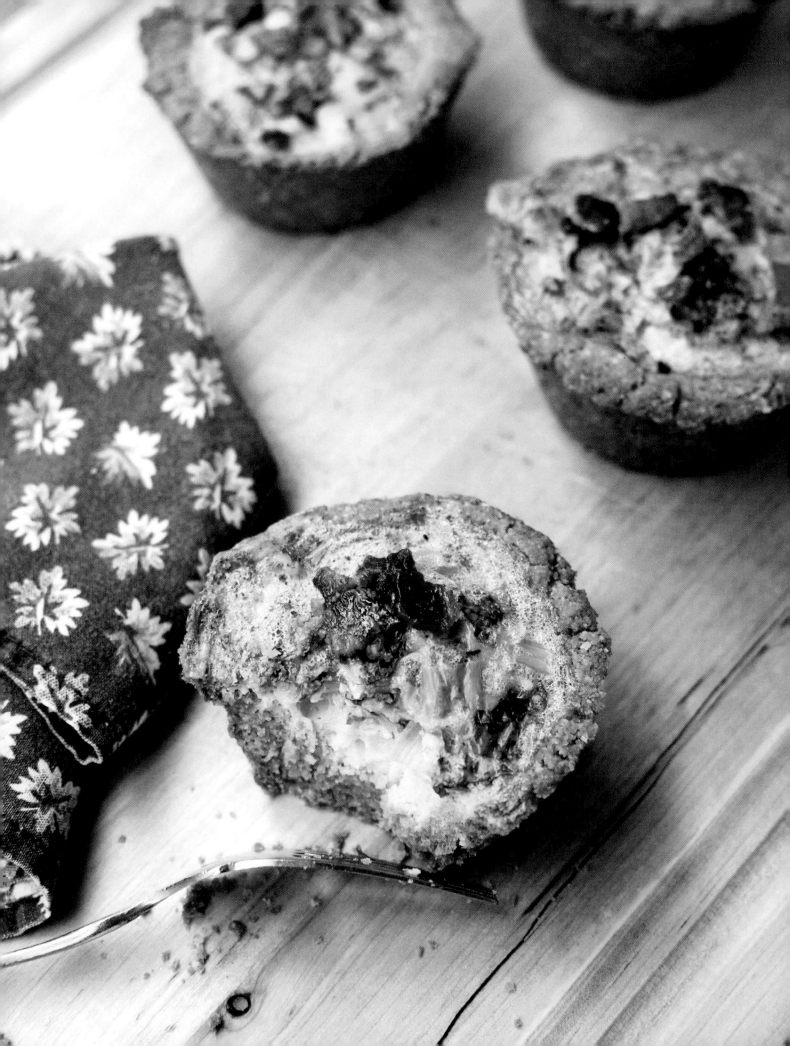

Banana-Pecan Pancakes

Makes about 15 pancakes
Dairy Free • Fish Free

1 cup (150 g) raw pecans

¼ cup (25 g) coconut flour, sifted

½ tsp baking soda

5 eggs

2 medium ripe bananas, mashed (about ½-⅔ cup)

1½ tsp pure vanilla extract

¾ tsp cinnamon

Pinch nutmeg

¼ cup (60 mL) coconut milk (full-fat or light, if needed)

This is basically your old favorite banana bread in the form of a pancake. I love the combo of sweet bananas and crunchy pecans and the fact that I can make a huge batch and freeze for quick midweek breakfasts for my kids. Just heat in a toaster oven or microwave, scramble an egg on the side, and you have a fast, delicious, healthy Paleo breakfast any kid would devour!

1. Place the pecans in a food processor and pulse until a fine meal is formed.

2. Place the ground pecans and the remaining ingredients, except the coconut milk, in a medium bowl and blend well with a hand mixer to combine. Tip: Add coconut milk only if the batter is too thick. Depending on the moisture level of the bananas I'm using, I don't always need it.

3. Drop ¼-cup scoops of batter onto a greased hot skillet. Cook until bubbling and browned on the edges, flip, and continue to cook until done, about 2 minutes per side.

4. Serve all by their lonesome or with a drizzle of pure maple syrup!

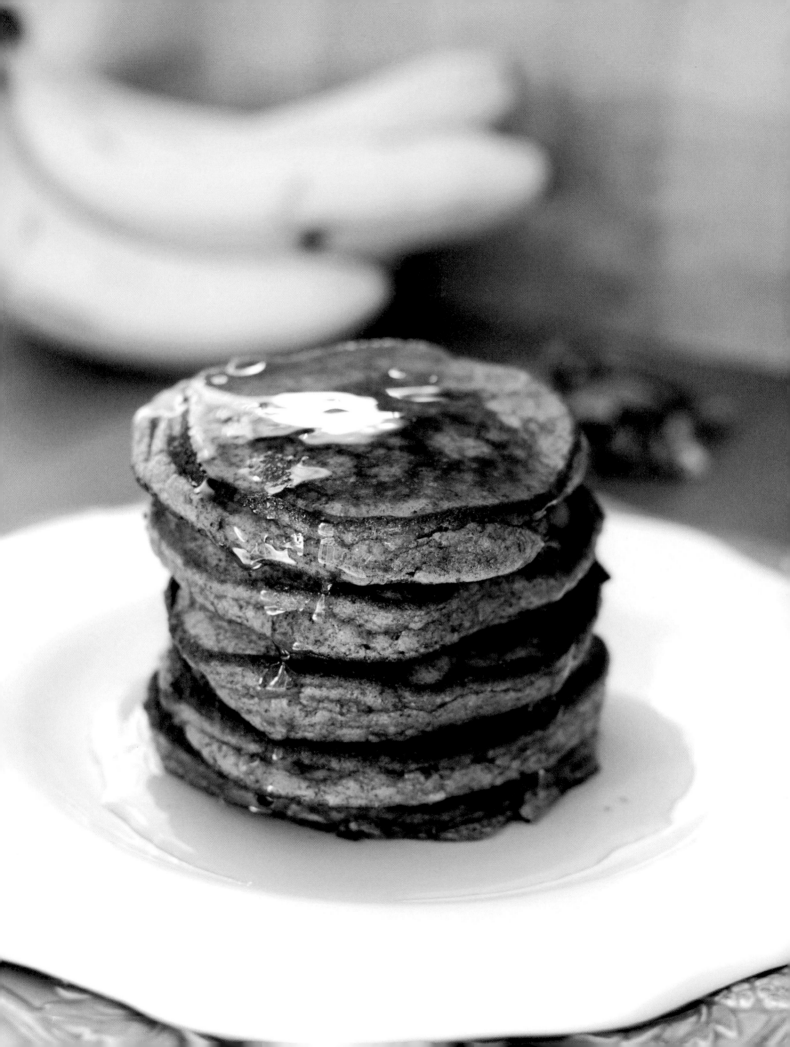

Gingerbread Pancakes with Cinnamon Syrup

Makes about 12 pancakes

Dairy Free • Fish Free

Dry Ingredients

¼ cup (30 g) almond flour

⅓ cup (35 g) coconut flour, sifted

½ tsp baking soda

Pinch sea salt

1½ tsp cinnamon

⅛ tsp nutmeg

¾ tsp ginger

Wet Ingredients

¼ cup (60 g) canned pumpkin purée

5 eggs

½ tsp pure vanilla extract

¼ cup (60 mL) coconut milk (full-fat or light)

Syrup

1 cup (240 mL) pure maple syrup

1 cinnamon stick (in a pinch you can use ½ tsp ground cinnamon)

These hearty, spicy pancakes are perfect for Christmas morning or a cold, snowy day. They make the house smell amazing, and they taste even better! The cinnamon syrup makes these pancakes even more special than they already are.

1. Place the dry ingredients in a medium bowl and whisk to combine.

2. Add the wet ingredients to the dry and blend with a hand mixer until completely smooth. The batter will be slightly thicker than traditional pancake batter, almost like a soft pudding.

3. Drop ¼-cup scoops of batter into a greased, hot skillet. Cook until bubbling and browned on the edges, flip, and continue to cook until done, about 2 minutes per side.

4. Meanwhile, make the syrup. Place the syrup ingredients in a small saucepan and heat over medium heat until bubbles start to form around the edges. Turn heat to low and keep warm until ready to serve, stirring occasionally to help infuse the syrup with that cinnamon flavor!

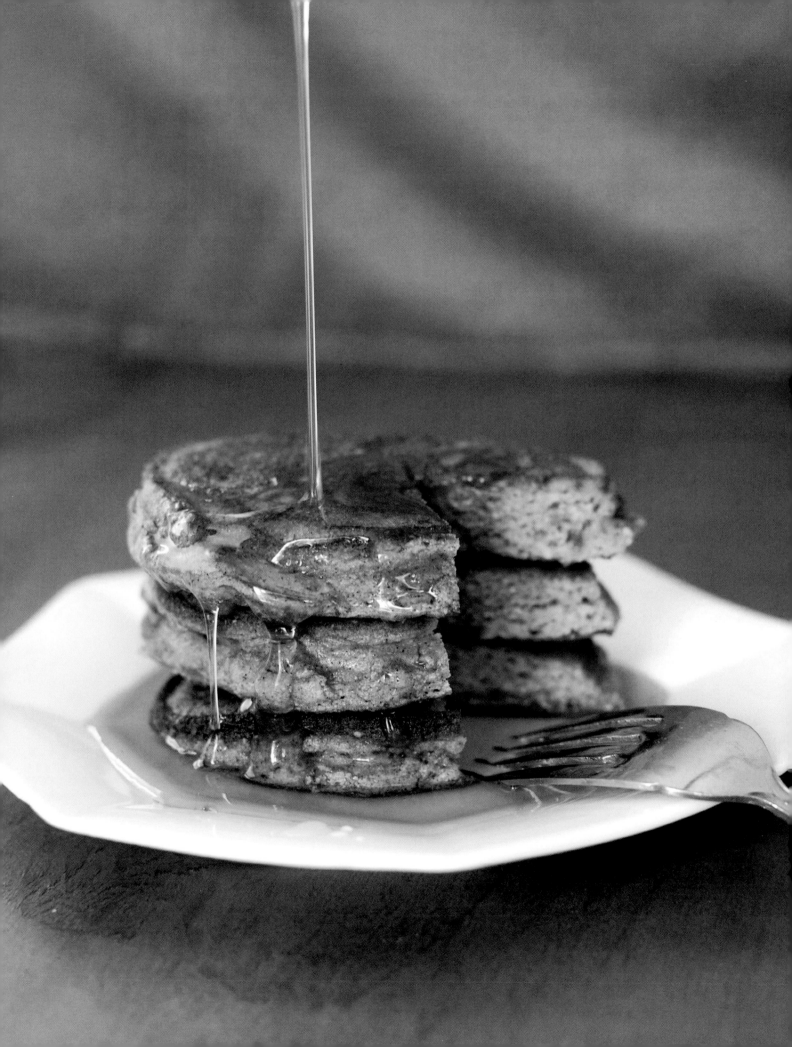

Bacon Guacamole

Makes about 2 cups

Dairy Free • Egg Free • Fish Free • Nut Free

1 large, ripe Hass avocado (or 2 medium)

5 strips cooked bacon, crumbled (US Wellness Meats)

2 tsp bacon drippings

1 roma tomato, diced

2 TBSP minced onion

1 garlic clove, minced

¼ tsp cumin

½ tsp chili powder

Sea salt and freshly ground black pepper to taste

Squeeze lime juice

Avocados are creamy, fatty goodness, and nutritional powerhouses to boot. Great on their own, but simply irresistible with the addition of a few spices and bacon. This dip is a family favorite for our annual Super Bowl party when served with veggie sticks and cooked bacon strips for dipping!

1. Place avocado flesh in a medium bowl and mash with a fork until fairly smooth.

2. Add the remaining ingredients and stir to combine.

3. Adjust seasonings to taste. Serve immediately.

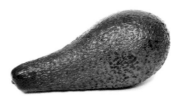

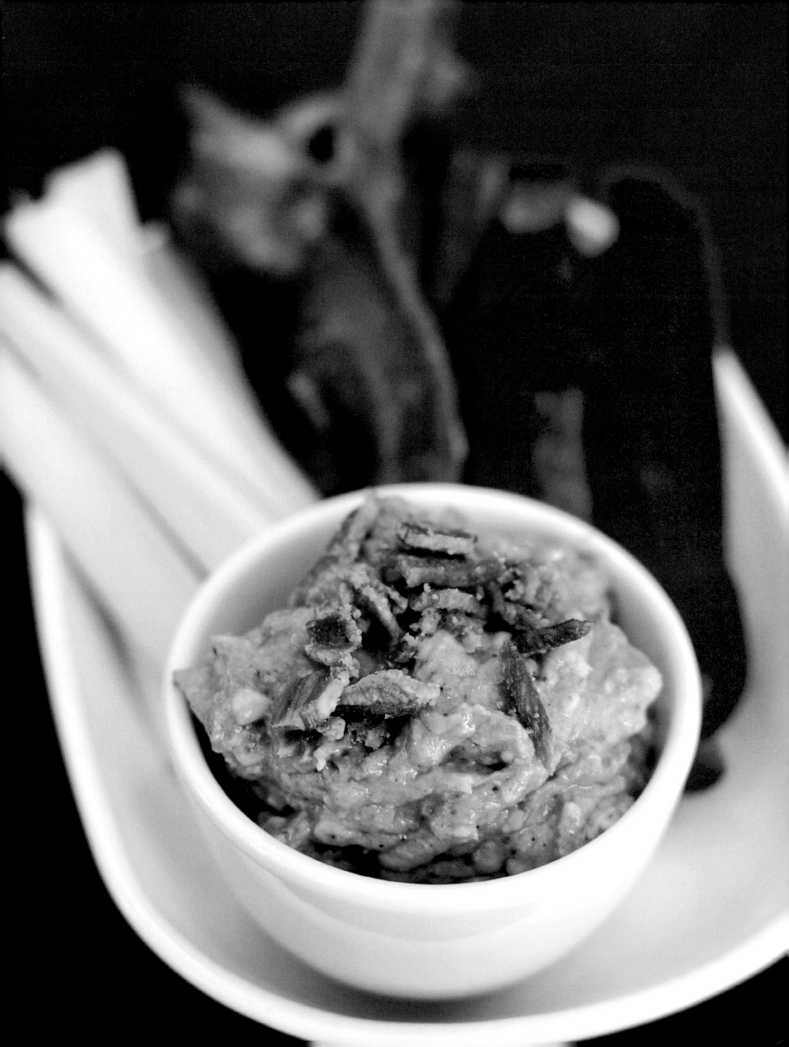

Pico de Gallo

Makes about 2 cups
Dairy Free • Egg Free • Fish Free • Nut Free

3-4 ripe roma tomatoes

1 medium jalapeño pepper

¼ cup (40 g) diced red onion

¼ cup (30 g) chopped cilantro

Squeeze lime juice

Sea salt and freshly ground black pepper to taste

I love this fresh salsa! We make it several times a week in the summer to pile on top of eggs or grilled steaks, chicken, or pork. It's a snap to make and packed with flavor. And you can adjust the few simple ingredients to really suit your taste. Love the spice? Don't discard the ribs or seeds from the jalapeño—that's where the heat is! Like onion? Use a whole one! And if cilantro really floats your boat, double or triple the amount. It's totally up to you!

1. Dice tomato. Place in a medium bowl.

2. Trim the end from the jalapeño. Cut in half lengthwise. With a spoon, remove the ribs and seeds and discard.

3. Dice the jalapeño and add to the tomatoes.

4. Add the onion and cilantro to the bowl.

5. Squeeze a little bit of lime juice on top, season with salt and pepper to taste, and stir to combine. Enjoy!

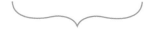

Note:
After a day or so, the tomatoes will look a little tired, so I toss the salsa into my food processor and process into a smooth-style salsa. It still tastes great and gets a fresh new look!

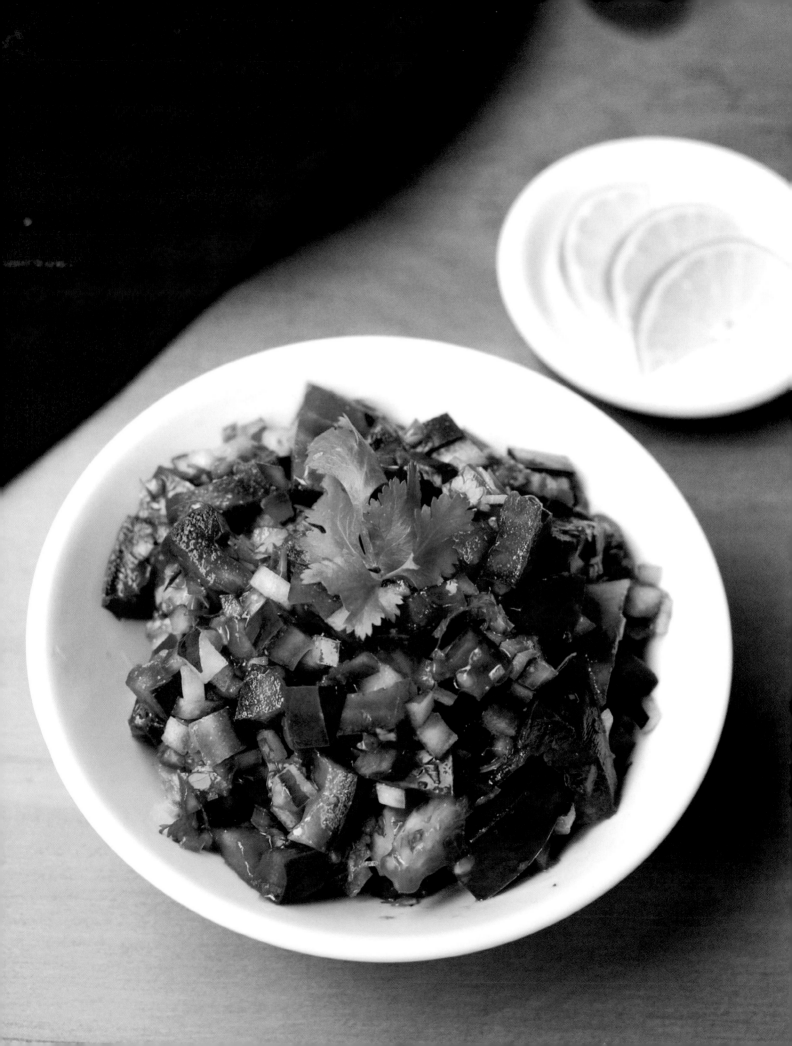

Onion Dip

Makes about 2½ cups
Egg Free • Nut Free

1 TBSP coconut oil

1 medium yellow onion, finely diced

8 oz (230 g) sour cream

1 tsp Worcestershire sauce

½ tsp granulated garlic

½ tsp sea salt

¼ tsp freshly ground black pepper

As I've mentioned, dairy is a personal choice in the world of Paleo. My family is o.k. with having a high-quality dairy indulgence a couple times a year and this delicious dip more than fits the bill! Say goodbye to that packet of soup mix—I'll take my onion dip without MSG, please! This recipe can be easily doubled for a crowd.

1. Heat the oil in a large skillet over medium heat. Add the onions and stir to coat. Cook the onions, stirring only occasionally, until they are cooked well, evenly browned and caramelized, about 30 minutes. Let them cool.

2. Place the remaining ingredients and onions in a medium bowl and stir well to mix.

3. Cover and refrigerate the dip overnight to let the flavors develop. Keeps up to 3 days in the fridge.

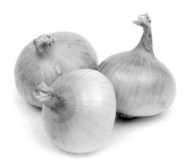

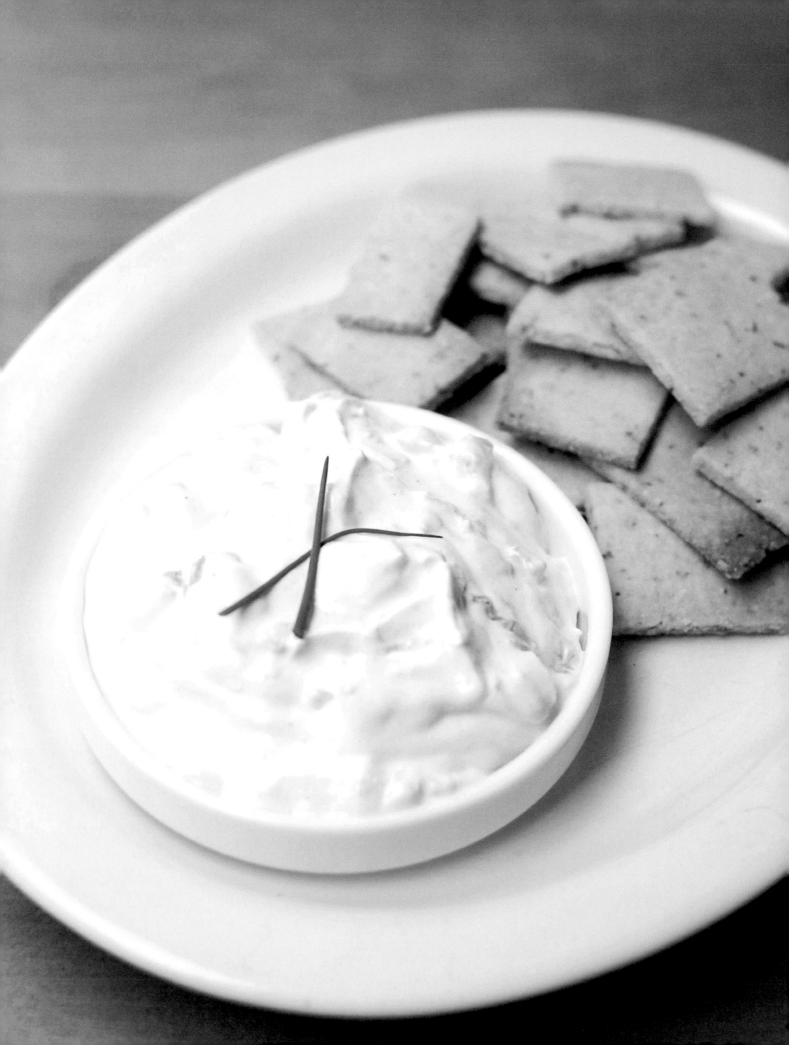

Bacon Dip

Makes about 2½ cups

Egg Free • Nut Free

1 TBSP coconut oil

1 medium yellow onion, finely diced

6 strips bacon, cooked and crumbled

2 TBSP reserved bacon grease

8 oz (230 g) sour cream

1 tsp Worcestershire sauce

½ tsp granulated garlic

¼ tsp smoked paprika

½ tsp sea salt

¼ tsp freshly ground black pepper

Bacon. Dip. 'Nuff said. Serve with cut-up veggies and tasty Seeded Crackers (page 108) or Italian Herb Crackers (page 106) for a satisfying game-night treat.

1. Heat the oil in a large skillet over medium heat. Add the onions and stir to coat. Cook the onions, stirring only occasionally, until they are cooked well, evenly browned, and caramelized, about 30 minutes. Let them cool.

2. Place the remaining ingredients and onions in a medium bowl and stir well to mix.

3. Cover and refrigerate the dip overnight to let the flavors develop. Keeps up to 3 days in the fridge.

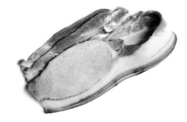

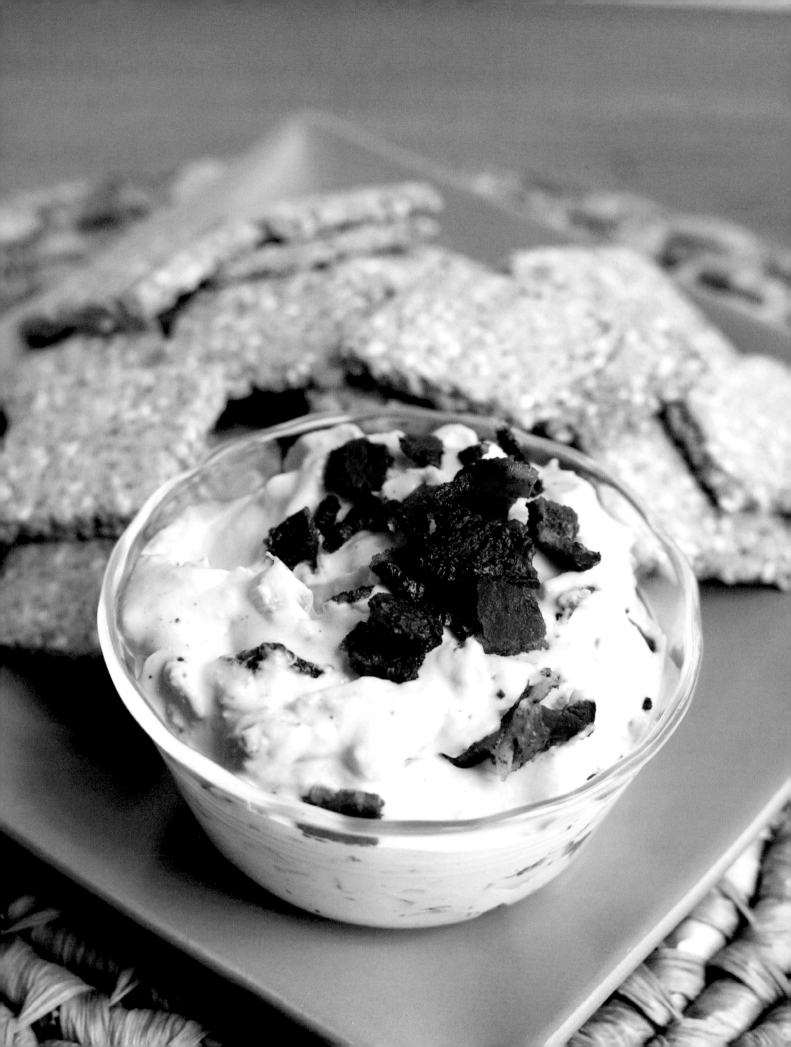

Roasted Sweet Potato Salad

Makes about 8 cups
Dairy Free • Fish Free • Nut Free

Potatoes

4-5 large sweet potatoes, peeled and cut into cubes

3 TBSP coconut oil, melted

1 tsp coarse sea salt

Freshly ground black pepper to taste

Salad

2-3 stalks celery, chopped

1 cup (190 g) diced carrots

¼ cup (40 g) diced red onion

1 5.75-oz (163 g) can black olives

1 TBSP chopped fresh dill (or 1 tsp dried)

1 TBSP chopped fresh parsley

⅓ cup (80 g) Paleo mayo, or more to taste (go to www.everydaypaleo.com for a great mayo recipe)

1 TBSP raw apple cider vinegar

1 tsp granulated onion

Sea salt and freshly ground black pepper to taste

This twist on a traditional potato salad will be a huge hit at your next potluck or picnic. Roasted sweet potatoes hold their shape wonderfully, and even the most diehard white potato fan will be won over by the burst of color.

1. Preheat the oven to 450°F.

2. Place the sweet potatoes in a large bowl, add the coconut oil, and stir to coat. Add salt and pepper to taste.

3. Place the sweet potatoes in an even layer on a parchment-lined baking sheet. Bake 20-25 minutes, or until potatoes are soft and browned. Cool in the pan on a wire rack.

4. Meanwhile, mix the salad ingredients in a large bowl. Add cooled sweet potatoes and stir to combine. Adjust seasonings to taste. Chill salad 1 hour before serving. Store salad in an airtight container in the fridge up to 2 days.

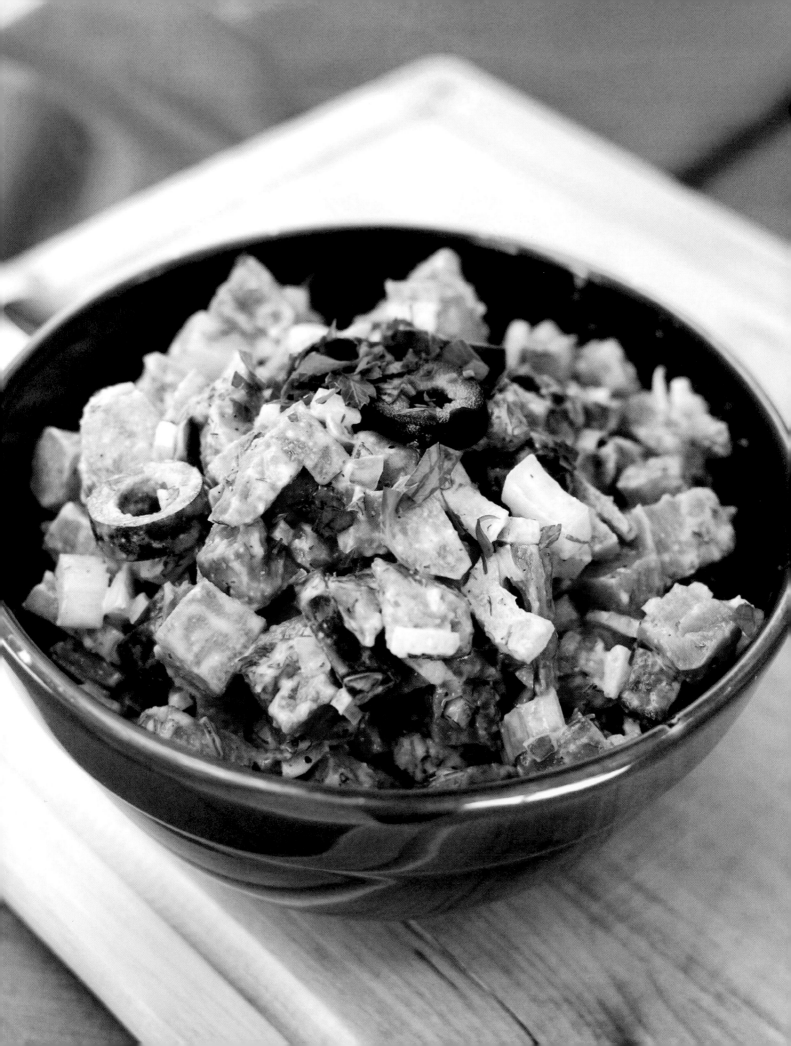

Garlic Kale Chips

Makes about 2 cups
Dairy Free* • Egg Free • Fish Free • Nut Free

Garlic Topping

2 TBSP coconut oil

2 TBSP ghee (or *2 more TBSP coconut oil, if you're going dairy-free)

2 garlic cloves, minced

⅛ tsp granulated garlic

Chips

1 bunch curly-leaf kale, stems removed, then washed, dried completely, and torn into bigger bite-size pieces

Sea salt

There are dozens of kale chip recipes on the Internet, but this garlicky one really kicks it up a notch. Kale chips are decadently crispy and melt in your mouth, so even kiddos happily scarf 'em up. And any time I can get my kids to inhale a nutritional megastar like kale, I'm happy too!

1. Preheat the oven to 350°F.

2. Place the topping ingredients in a small saucepan over low heat for 2-3 minutes to warm. Remove from the heat and set aside to cool about 10 minutes.

3. Place the kale in a large bowl. Pour the topping over it.

4. With your fingers, gently rub the oil into the leaves, making sure all are coated with oil.

5. Place the kale in a single layer on a parchment-lined baking sheet.

6. Bake 12-15 minutes, rotating tray partway through, until kale is crispy but still green. Watch it carefully those last few minutes, as it can turn dark brown quickly, resulting in slightly bitter chips.

7. Sprinkle with sea salt and enjoy!

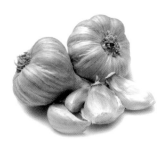

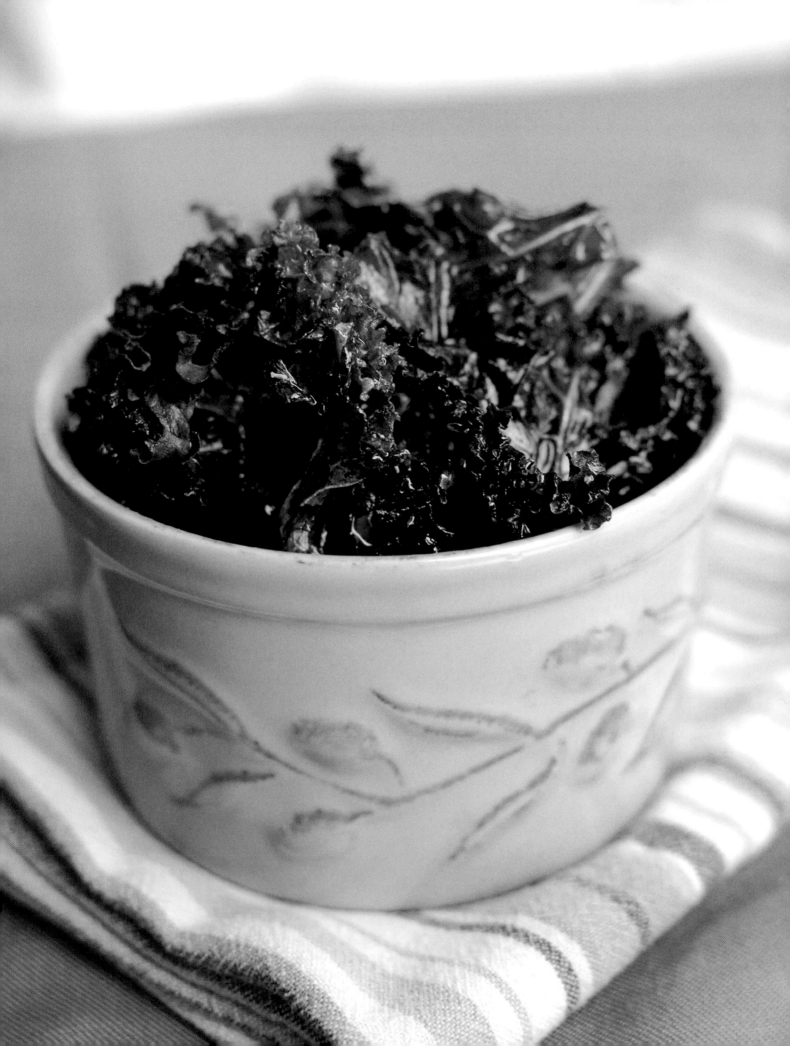

Onion Rings

Makes enough to coat 2 whole onions
Dairy Free • Fish Free

¼ cup (30 g) almond flour

2 TBSP coconut flour, sifted

¼ cup (30 g) arrowroot starch

¼ tsp paprika

½ tsp granulated garlic

⅛ tsp turmeric

½ tsp granulated onion

2 eggs

⅓-½ cup (80-120 mL) coconut milk (full-fat or light)

Coconut oil for frying

2 large yellow onions, sliced into thin rings

Let's face it, fried foods, even if gluten-free or Paleo, are not the healthiest option. But even folks following a Paleo lifestyle occasionally miss having a "normal" restaurant item like onion rings. And it's impossible to satisfy that craving at a restaurant: Wheat flour? Bread crumbs? Rancid oil? That sounds appetizing. So when we want a "restaurant night out," we treat ourselves at home, where we know that all the ingredients are organic, high quality, fresh, and, most of all, safe. I highly advise eating fried foods only occasionally, but enjoy every bite when you do, then lose the guilt and move on.

1. Place the flours, arrowroot, paprika, garlic, turmeric, and onion in a medium bowl and whisk to combine.

2. Add the eggs and ⅓ cup coconut milk. Whisk until smooth. If the batter is too thick, add additional coconut milk for desired consistency.

3. In a large non-stick skillet, heat enough oil to come half way up the sides of the onion slices to 330°F. It's best to use a thermometer to ensure proper oil temperature.

4. Coat onion slices in batter, tapping off excess, and place gently in hot oil. Cook for about 2 minutes per side, or until golden brown. Repeat until all onions are cooked, adding additional oil to the pan if necessary.

5. Use tongs to remove cooked onions to a paper-towel-lined tray, sprinkle with sea salt if desired, and serve immediately.

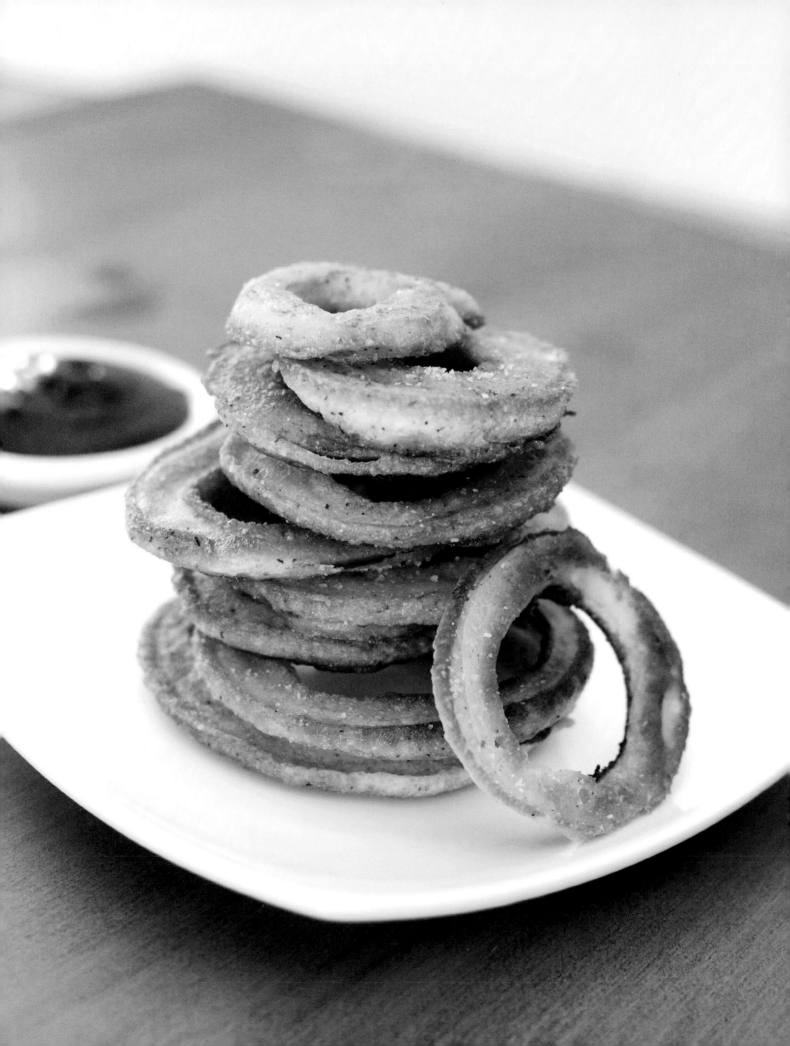

Sweet Potato Fries
with Garlic Oil

Makes about 2½ cups
Dairy Free • Egg Free • Fish Free • Nut Free

Fries

2 medium sweet potatoes,
peeled and cut into French
fries

1 TBSP sea salt

2 TBSP coconut oil, melted

Freshly ground black pepper

Garlic Oil

2 TBSP extra-virgin olive oil

2 garlic cloves, minced

Oven-baked sweet potatoes take on new life with the addition of crispy little garlic bits! At first glance this recipe may seem to call for a lot of salt, but keep in mind that salt draws water out of the potatoes, which helps them crisp up in the oven. Plus, you'll be washing off most of the salt before baking so you won't be consuming all of it.

1. Preheat the oven to 450°F.

2. Place the sweet potatoes in a colander, sprinkle with salt, and let drain about 20 minutes.

3. Rinse the sweet potatoes thoroughly with cold water. Pat dry with a towel and really squeeze the potatoes to help pull out any extra moisture.

4. Place the fries in a medium bowl, add the coconut oil and pepper and toss to coat.

5. Place the fries on a greased baking sheet in a single layer without touching and bake for 20-25 minutes, or until cooked through and browned, turning fries once to brown evenly.

6. Meanwhile, make the garlic oil. Heat a small saucepan over low heat. Add the oil and minced garlic. Cook until garlic is just starting to turn golden. Remove from heat.

7. Place cooked fries in the medium bowl, pour garlic oil over them, and toss to coat.

8. Serve with Fry Sauce (page 140).

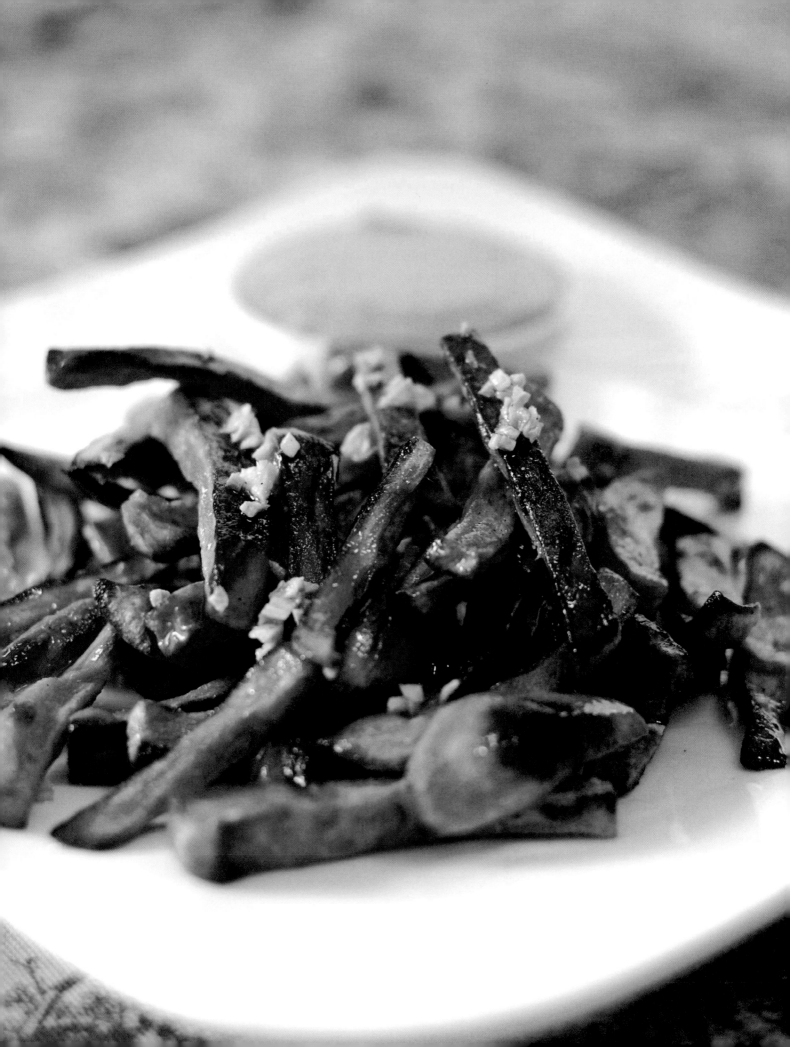

Fry Sauce

Makes about ¾ cup

Dairy Free • Fish Free • Nut Free

2 TBSP Paleo mayo (go to www.everydaypaleo.com for recipe)

¼ cup (60 mL) ketchup (go to www.paleocomfortfoods. com for recipe)

1 clove garlic, sliced

1 TBSP olive oil

1 tsp raw apple cider vinegar (or lemon juice)

2 TBSP finely chopped yellow onion

1 tsp yellow mustard

Pinch cayenne pepper (or more if you like it spicy)

Sea salt and freshly ground black pepper to taste

My favorite drive-in hamburger restaurant—yes they still exist—serves up a fry sauce that is even better than the fries themselves! Here's my version, without the added sugar and preservatives. This sauce works for sweet potato fries and hamburgers, and we even enjoy it on uncured, grass-fed beef hot dogs on occasion! To make this sauce less labor intensive, it's ok to purchase the highest quality, pre-made mayo and ketchup you can find. I promise, the world will not come to an end because you didn't make them from scratch!

1. Place all the ingredients in a food processor or blender and purée until mostly smooth, with only a few small bits remaining.

2. Serve with Sweet Potato Fries (page 138) or slather on your favorite burger!

Note:
Try adding a dash or two of your favorite hot sauce or chili paste for an extra kick!

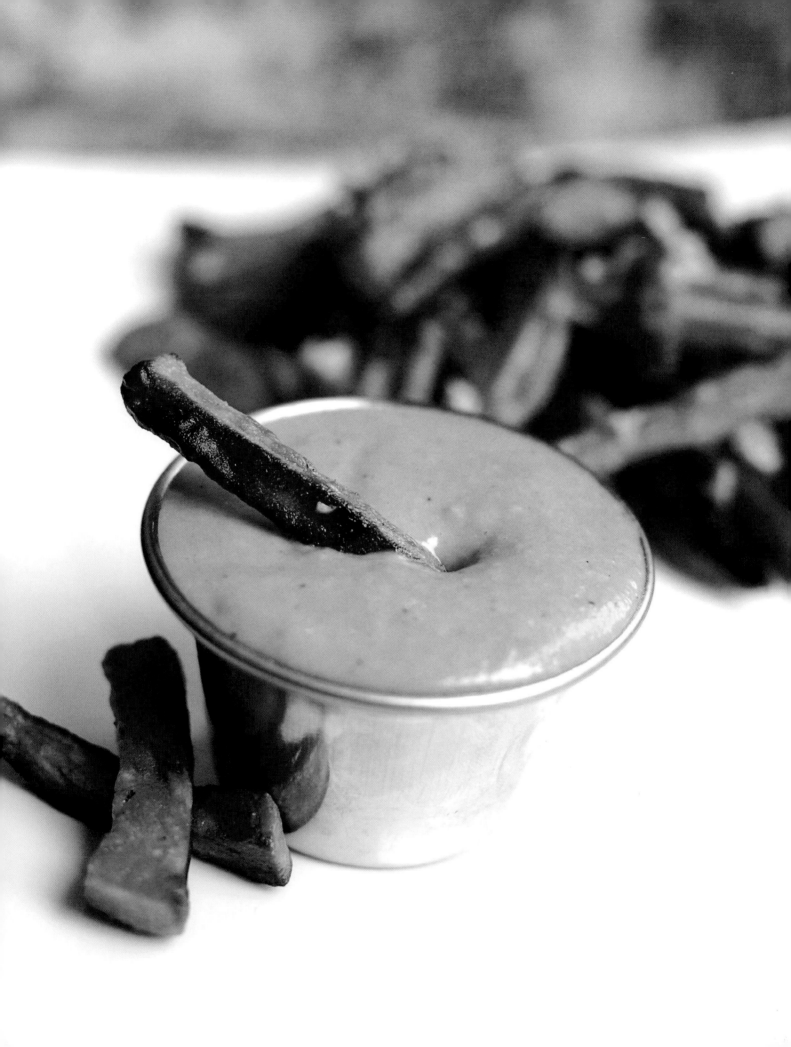

Hot Wings

Makes 4 servings

Dairy Free • Egg Free • Fish Free • Nut Free

Seasoning

1 TBSP paprika

2 tsp granulated onion

½ tsp granulated garlic

¼ tsp smoked paprika

1 tsp sea salt

Pinch rosemary

Freshly ground black pepper to taste

Wings

3 lbs (1,350 g) chicken drumettes, washed and patted dry (US Wellness Meats)

2 TBSP coconut oil

Sauce

1 15-oz (420 g) can tomato sauce

1 6-oz (168 g) can tomato paste

¼ cup (40 g) diced yellow onion

3 garlic cloves, minced

3 TBSP pure maple syrup or raw honey

3 TBSP raw apple cider vinegar

2 tsp sea salt

1 tsp paprika

½ tsp smoked paprika

1 TBSP coconut aminos

Pinch cayenne (or more if you like it spicy)

Restaurant wings are loaded with gluten and fried in rancid vegetable oil. Thanks, but no thanks. Wings are delicious and oh-so easy to make, so who needs a restaurant anyway? This recipe makes lots of sauce, and the leftover is prefect over meatballs or spooned on top of meatloaf. You can also freeze extra sauce for the next time you get a hankering for wings!

1. Preheat the oven to 375°F.

2. Mix the seasoning ingredients together in a small bowl.

3. Place the wings in a large bowl and coat with oil. Sprinkle seasoning over wings and rub in evenly with your hands. Don't forget to wash your hands now!

4. Line a large baking sheet with aluminum foil. Grease the foil. Place the wings evenly on the foil, keeping them from touching so they bake evenly and crisply.

5. Place the wings in the oven and bake 30 minutes, then turn oven up to 450°F and bake 20 minutes more, until wings are browned, crispy, and cooked through.

6. Meanwhile, combine all the sauce ingredients in a large saucepan over medium-low heat until heated through.

7. Place cooked wings in a large bowl, add enough sauce to make yourself happy, and toss lightly to evenly coat wings. Devour! Don't forget the napkins!

Note:
Add as much of your favorite hot sauce to the sauce mixture as you like!

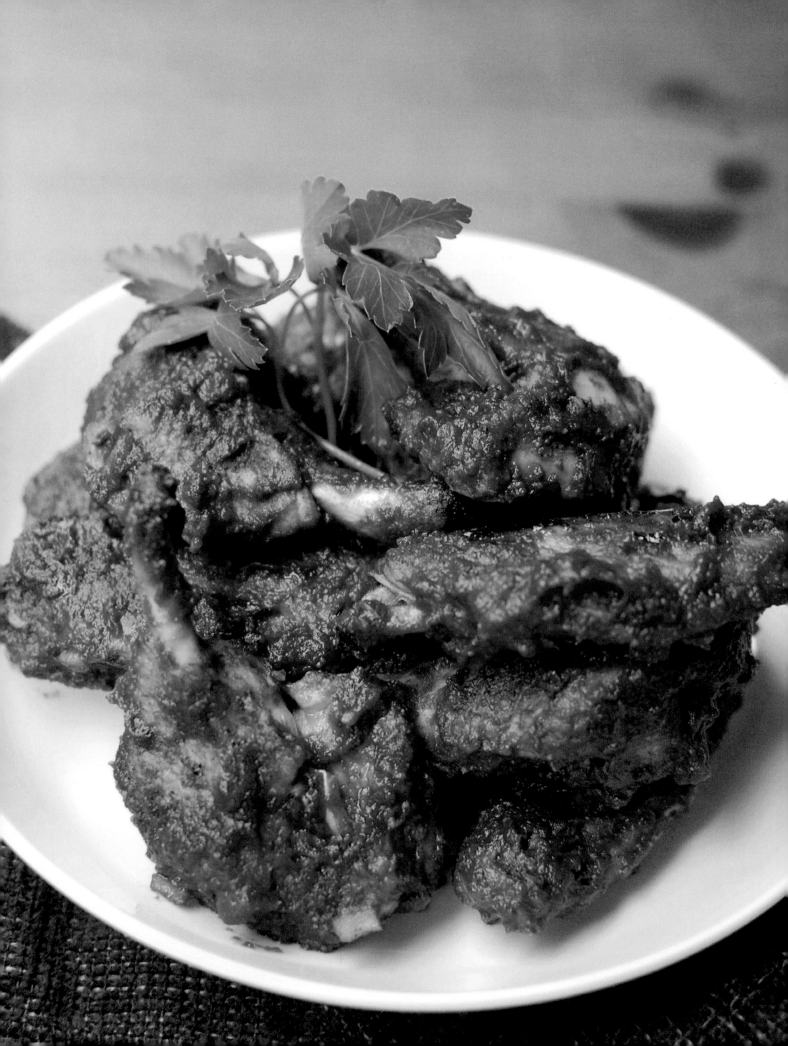

Cincinnati Chili

Makes 4 to 6 servings
Dairy Free • Egg Free • Nut Free

2 TBSP coconut oil

1 large onion, chopped

1 lb (450 g) ground beef (US Wellness Meats)

3 cloves garlic, minced

1 TBSP chili powder

½ tsp allspice

1 tsp cinnamon

1 tsp cumin

¼ tsp cayenne pepper (more or less to taste)

½ tsp sea salt

2 tsp paprika

⅛ tsp cloves

1½ TBSP unsweetened cocoa powder

1 15-oz (420 g) can tomato sauce

1 TBSP Worcestershire sauce

1 TBSP raw apple cider vinegar

1 cup (240 mL) water

Cincinnati chili is a regional style of chili con carne with typically un-chili-like seasonings, such as cinnamon, cloves, allspice, and chocolate. Another twist is that it's usually served over spaghetti! I love making this uniquely flavored chili when I need a hot, filling bowl of goodness to take the chill off winter. I put my own Paleo twist on it by serving it over cooked spaghetti squash and top it with diced onions or chopped green onions!

1. Heat the oil in a stockpot. Add the onion and cook 2 minutes over medium heat.

2. Add the ground beef, garlic, and chili powder and cook until the meat is browned and no longer pink.

3. Add the remaining ingredients, stirring to combine. Bring to a simmer. Reduce heat to low and simmer, uncovered, for 1½ hours.

4. Serve as is or over cooked spaghetti squash!

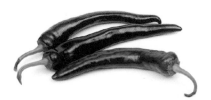

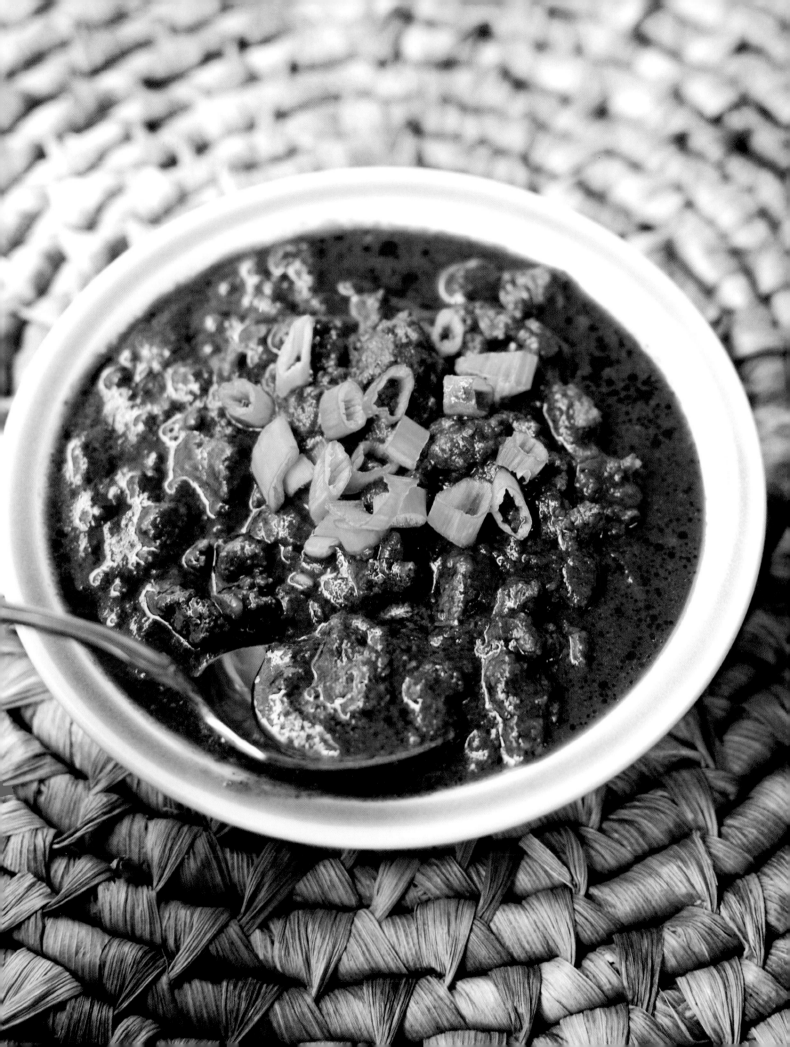

Chicken 'n Dumplings

Makes 4 to 6 servings

Dairy Free • Fish Free • Nut Free

Chicken

2 TBSP coconut oil

1 small yellow onion, diced

2 garlic cloves, minced

1 8-oz (230 g) package white mushrooms, sliced

1 cup (150 g) diced celery

1 cup (150 g) diced carrots

1 cup (150 g) diced parsnips

1 cup (150 g) diced zucchini

2 lbs (900 g) boneless skinless chicken breasts (or thighs), cubed (US Wellness Meats)

¼ cup (40 g) chopped fresh parsley

1 tsp chopped fresh rosemary

1 tsp chopped fresh sage

6 cups (1.425 L) homemade chicken broth

Sea salt and freshly ground black pepper to taste

Dumplings

⅓ cup (35 g) coconut flour, sifted

½ tsp baking powder

¼ tsp sea salt

4 eggs

3 TBSP coconut oil, melted

Chicken and dumplings just spell c-o-m-f-o-r-t. My mom used to make them on cold winter days when I was growing up, and they always filled me with warmth and a sense of home. I knew I needed to have a Paleo version of this dish to keep those memories alive, and I'm so glad I did. You'll feel like mom's right there with you when you sit down to this classic meal!

1. Make the chicken: Heat the oil in a large stockpot over medium heat. Add the onion and garlic. Cook 2 minutes.

2. Add the mushrooms, celery, carrots, parsnips, and zucchini. Cook 5 minutes. Remove to a plate and keep warm.

3. Add the chicken to the stockpot. Cook until done, stirring occasionally, about 6-7 minutes.

4. Add the veggies back to pot. Add the parsley, rosemary, sage, and chicken stock. Season with salt and pepper and simmer for 10 minutes.

5. Make the dumplings: Place all the dumpling ingredients in a small bowl and stir well to mix.

6. Drop spoonfuls of dumpling dough into the simmering pot. Cover, turn heat to medium-low, and cook 20 minutes, or until dumplings are cooked through. Serve!

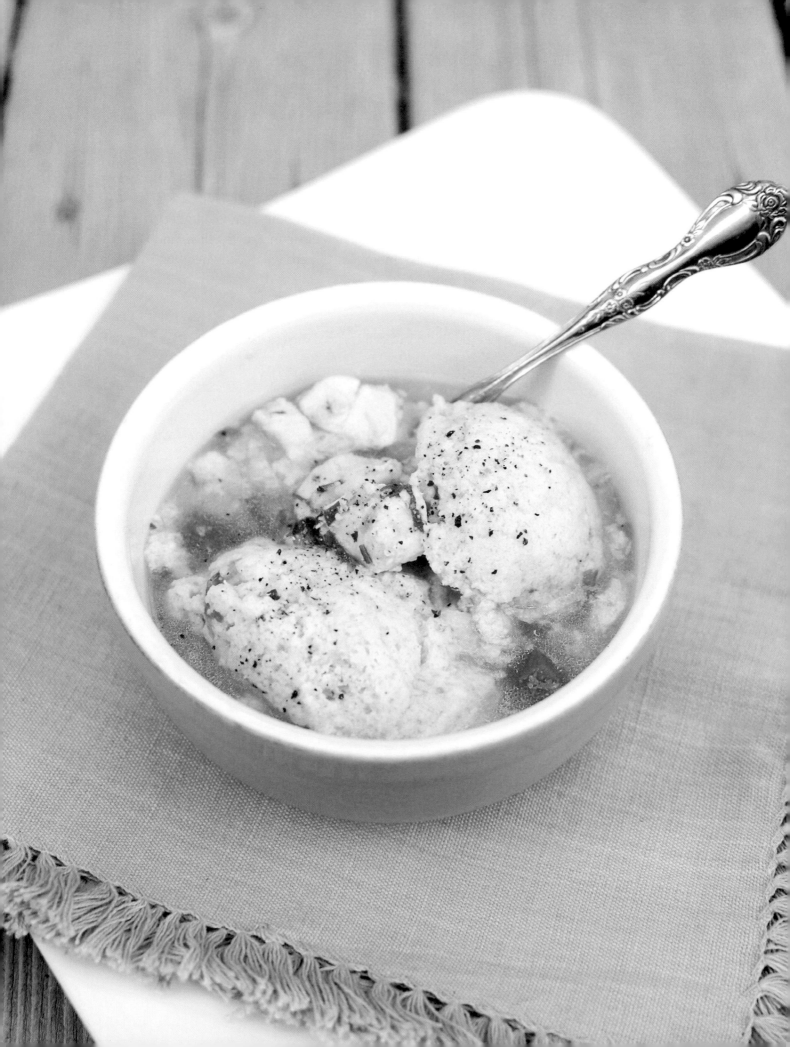

Bacon Burger

Makes 4 servings

Dairy Free • Egg Free • Nut Free

1 lb (450 g) ground beef (US Wellness Meats)

4-6 strips cooked bacon (not crispy), chopped

¼ cup (40 g) finely minced onion

2 tsp Worcestershire sauce

½ tsp rosemary

¼ tsp smoked paprika

1 garlic clove, minced

Freshly ground black pepper to taste

Maple Pancake Buns (recipe follows)

I know lots of people like bacon piled on their burgers, but honestly? It's kind of hard to bite off some bacon without destroying your burger. So I decided to add it to the burger itself, which means bite-size pieces of bacon with every mouthful! Oh, and did I mention the maple pancake "buns" to help you corral all the bacon-y goodness? Giddy up!

1. Place the first 8 ingredients in a medium bowl and mix to combine.

2. Shape into 4 patties.

3. Grill or cook the patties in a greased cast-iron skillet until browned on both sides and cooked to medium, about 4-5 minutes per side.

4. Serve with your favorite toppings on Maple Pancake Buns.

Maple Pancake Buns

Dry Ingredients

¼ cup (30 g) almond flour

3 TBSP coconut flour, sifted

Pinch sea salt

½ tsp baking powder

Wet Ingredients

4 eggs

½ tsp pure vanilla extract

2 TBSP pure maple syrup

2 TBSP coconut oil, melted, plus more for greasing

1. Place the dry ingredients in a medium bowl and whisk to combine.

2. Add the wet ingredients, except the oil. Blend slightly.

3. Add the oil and mix well. Let the batter sit 2-3 minutes to thicken.

4. Drop ¼-cup scoops of batter onto a greased hot skillet. Cook until bubbling and browned on the edges, flip, and continue to cook until done, about 2 minutes per side.

5. Cool slightly. Ready to use as hamburger buns—or for a breakfast treat!

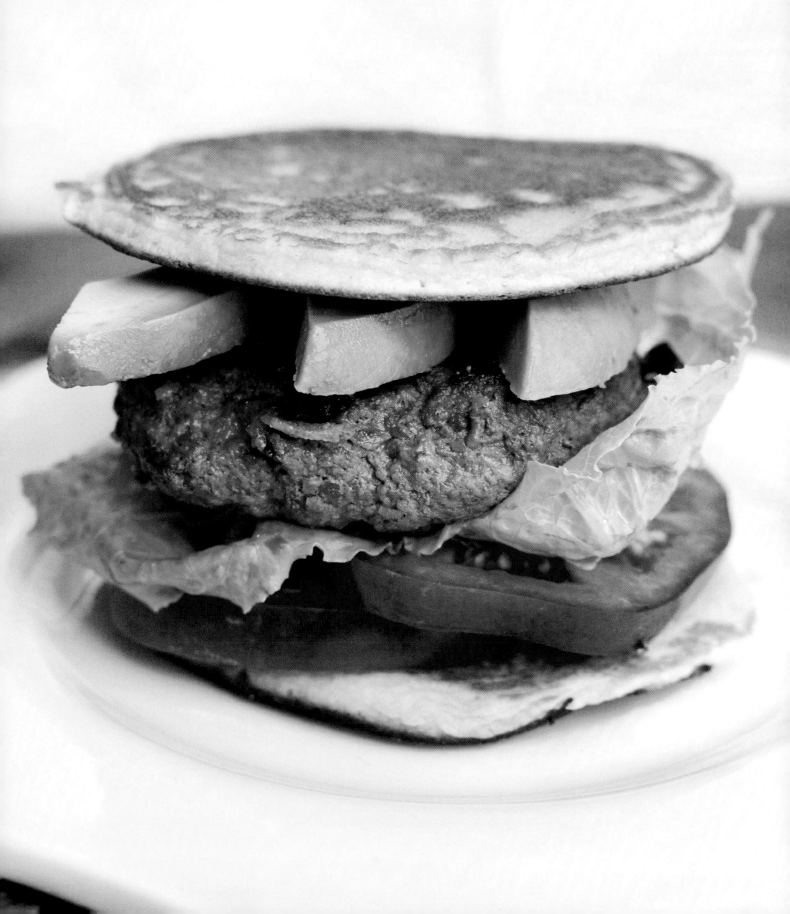

Rosemary Pork Burgers

Makes 4 servings

Dairy Free • Egg Free • Fish Free • Nut Free

1 lb (450 g) ground pork (US Wellness Meats)

½ tsp chopped fresh rosemary

½ tsp chopped fresh thyme

Sea salt and freshly ground black pepper to taste

¼ cup (40 g) finely chopped yellow onion

1 tsp Dijon mustard

½ cup (75 g) chopped fresh spinach

Sometimes we get tired of ground beef. Don't get me wrong—it's wonderful and all, especially since it's the most reasonably priced form of grass-fed meat. But that's also why we eat it A LOT. This tasty pork burger is still affordable but provides an unexpected taste and texture you just don't get in a traditional hamburger. A true dinner lifesaver!

1. Place all the ingredients in a medium bowl and mix to combine.

2. Form into 4 patties.

3. Grill the patties or cook in a greased cast-iron skillet over medium heat until browned and cooked through, about 5 minutes per side.

4. Top with your favorite garnishes: lettuce, tomatoes, avocado, grilled onions, pickles, kraut!

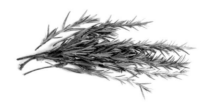

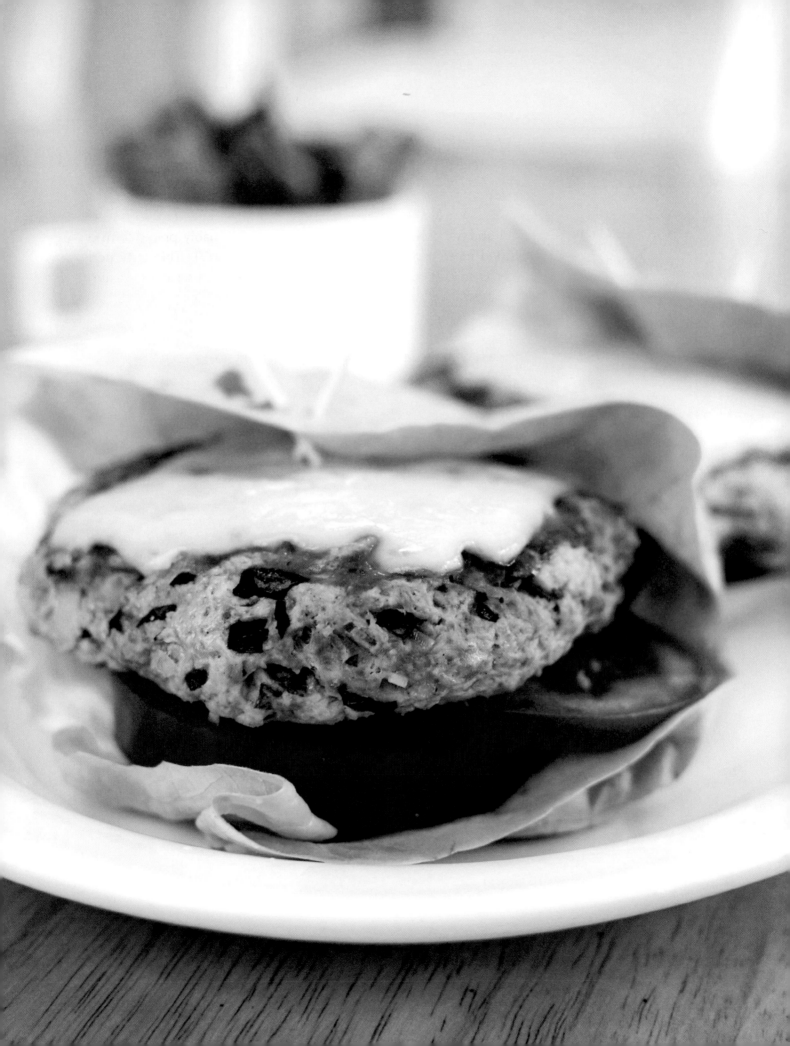

Slow-Cooker BBQ Beef

Makes 4 to 6 servings

Dairy Free • Egg Free • Fish Free • Nut Free

Beef

3-5 lbs (1,350-2,250 g) beef chuck roast (US Wellness Meats)

Sauce

1 15-oz (420 g) can tomato sauce

1 6-oz (168 g) can tomato paste

3 TBSP raw honey

2 TBSP raw apple cider vinegar

2 tsp sea salt

½ medium yellow onion, diced

3 garlic cloves, minced

1 tsp paprika

½ tsp smoked paprika

1 TBSP coconut aminos

1 tsp Liquid Smoke (see "Resources")

1 tsp oregano

⅛ tsp cayenne

Freshly ground black pepper to taste

Add Ons

Shredded lettuce

Red onion, diced

Chopped dill pickles (see "Resources")

Nothing goes together quite like a grass-fed beef roast, a slow cooker, and homemade barbecue sauce! I like to take shortcuts in the kitchen, so I don't usually brown the roast before placing it in the slow cooker, but feel free to add that step if it goes against your culinary sensibility to do otherwise. I won't be offended—I promise!

1. Place the roast in a large slow cooker.

2. Place all the sauce ingredients in a medium bowl and stir well to combine. Pour the sauce over the roast. Cover and cook on low 6-8 hours or until meat falls apart easily.

3. Shred beef in the pot using two forks. Serve over cooked spaghetti squash and top with diced red onions and chopped pickles!

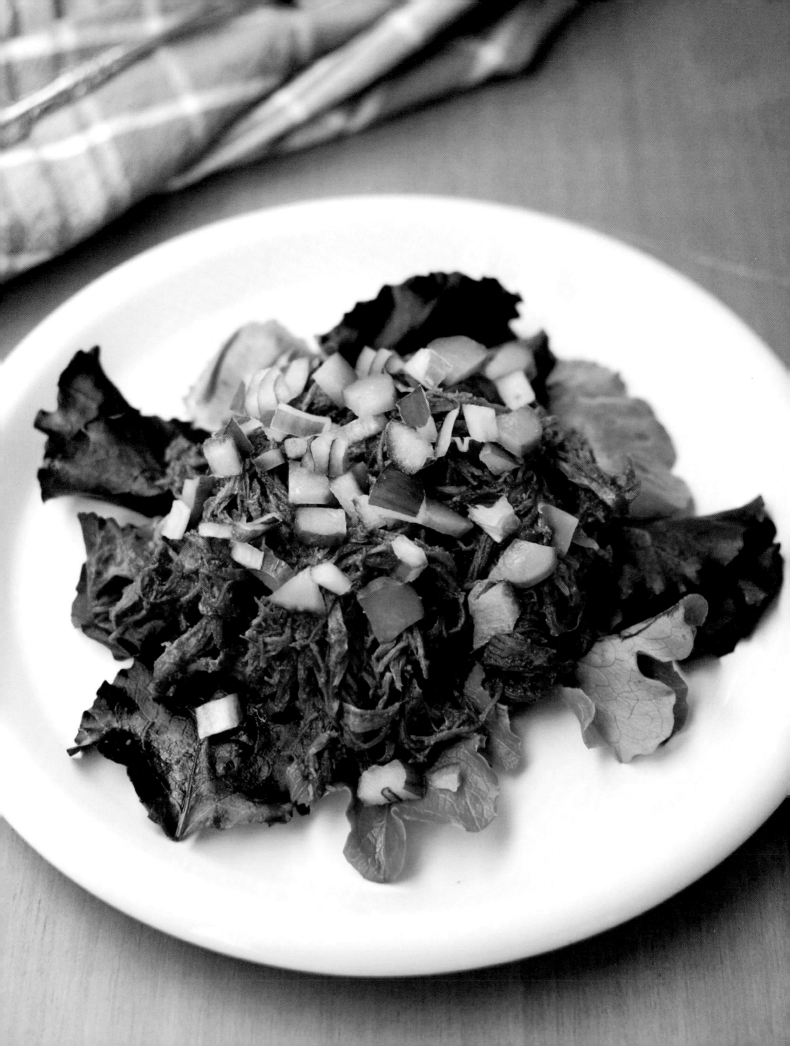

Paleo Fish Sticks

Makes 4 servings
Dairy Free • Egg Free

Coating

½ cup (75 g) raw macadamia nuts

½ cup (45 g) unsweetened finely shredded coconut

¼ tsp freshly ground black pepper

⅛ tsp turmeric

½ tsp granulated onion

½ tsp paprika

¼ tsp sea salt

Fish

1-2 lbs (900 g) firm white fish fillets or chicken, cut into small strips

Coconut oil for the pan

It's hard to get a lot of grain-free crumb coatings to stick to chicken or fish, but not this one! The lovely fat in the macadamias provides just enough moisture to keep everything put. Plus, the crust is thick, crunchy, AND nutritious. Try it on chicken strips too!

1. Place the macadamia nuts in a food processor and pulse into a fine meal.

2. Place the macadamia meal and the remaining coating ingredients in a shallow dish and mix to combine.

3. Rinse the fish in cold water and do not pat dry. You want it damp, but not soaked.

4. Toss each fish strip in the coating, using your fingers to help it stick.

5. Heat a nonstick skillet over medium-high heat. Melt enough coconut oil to cover the bottom and come partway up the sides of the fish. You don't want to deep-fry it; you need just enough oil to cook the fish evenly.

6. Brown the fish in the hot oil, flip, and brown the other side, about 3 minutes per side. Make sure you turn the fish only once! Continually flipping the fish will cause the coating to fall off, so commit to one flip after the fish is good and browned.

7. Place the cooked fish on a wire rack over a baking sheet while remaining fish cooks. Serve and enjoy!

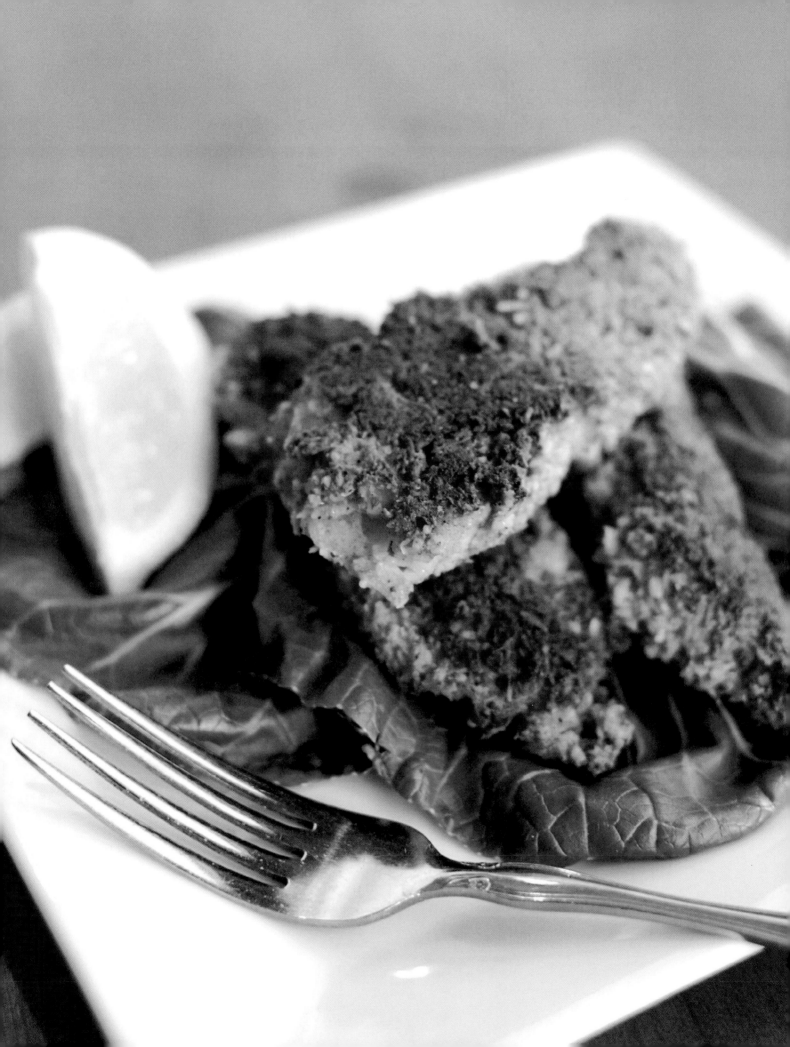

Meatball Sub

Dairy Free • Egg Free* • Fish Free

Meatballs

1 lb (450 g) ground beef (US Wellness Meats)

1 lb (450 g) ground pork (US Wellness Meats)

½ medium onion, finely chopped

3 garlic cloves, minced

¼ cup (40 g) chopped fresh parsley

½ tsp sea salt

1 tsp oregano

½ tsp basil

Pinch rosemary

½ tsp freshly ground black pepper

2 TBSP coconut flour, sifted

2 TBSP almond meal

2 TBSP extra-virgin olive oil, plus more for the pan

Super-Quick Bread (page 42)

Zucchini Pizza Boat sauce (page 162)

The meatballs in this dish are fantastic on their own and make a great appetizer for parties. But every so often I miss those meatball subs, with that bread soaking up some of the sauce. Oh, my. … Sorry, I was lost there for a moment. Anyway, instead of heading to my local sandwich shop and getting glutened up, I made my own version to satisfy that saucy yearning.

1. Place all the meatball ingredients in a medium bowl and mix lightly with your hands to combine.

2. Roll into 1½-inch balls.

3. Heat some olive oil in a large skillet over medium-high heat. Add the meatballs, spacing evenly around pan. Make sure not to touch them for a few minutes and really let them brown and caramelize on the bottoms. Brown bottoms are good bottoms! Turn meatballs to brown on all sides, lowering heat to medium if necessary.

4. Meanwhile, make the Super-Quick Bread and thaw out (and warm) some Zucchini Pizza Boat sauce. (Which I know you have in your freezer, right?)

5. Place meatballs in long dishes or bowls and spoon sauce over them. Cut quick bread in half and place alongside. Enjoy!!

Note:
* Egg-free if you omit the bread

Freeze any leftover meatballs for later use.

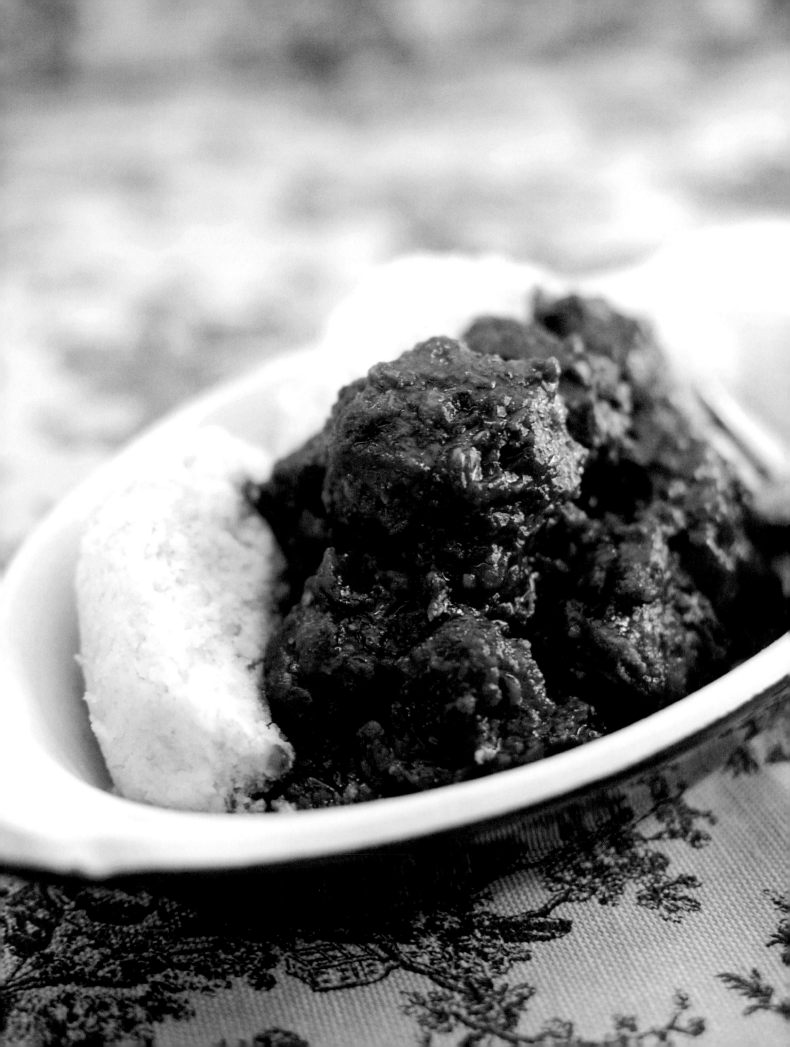

Salisbury Steak with Mushroom Gravy

Makes 4 servings

Dairy Free • Egg Free • Fish Free • Nut Free

Steaks

1½ lbs (680 g) ground beef
(US Wellness Meats)

½ medium yellow onion,
finely chopped

1 clove garlic, minced

2 tsp granulated onion

½ tsp chopped fresh
rosemary

1 tsp paprika

1 tsp fennel seed

1 tsp sea salt

Freshly ground black pepper
to taste

2 TBSP coconut oil

Gravy

8 oz (230 g) white
mushrooms, chopped

Sea salt and freshly ground
black pepper to taste

2 cups (475 mL) beef broth

½ cup (120 mL) coconut milk
(full-fat or light)

1 TBSP coconut flour, sifted

1 TBSP arrowroot starch
mixed with a tiny bit of cold
water to make a slurry

TV dinners have nothing on this delicious, hearty, and satisfying Salisbury steak! Well, except excessive sodium, and sugar, and preservatives, and trans-fats, and things I can't pronounce. Trust me, both your body and your taste buds will be better off with this version.

1. Place all the steak ingredients, except the coconut oil, in a medium bowl and mix gently to combine.

2. Form 4 large oval patties, about 1-inch thick.

3. Heat the coconut oil in a large nonstick skillet over medium-high heat and add the patties.

4. Cook until browned and caramelized, about 6 minutes per side.

5. Remove the patties to a platter and keep warm by tenting with foil.

6. Make the gravy. Add the mushrooms to the pan. Season with salt and pepper and cook until tender, about 5 minutes.

7. Add the beef broth and coconut milk to pan.

8. Add the coconut flour and stir. Bring to a boil.

9. Add the arrowroot slurry and stir until thick, about 1 minute. Remove gravy from heat.

10. Serve Salisbury steaks with mushroom gravy ladled over the top!

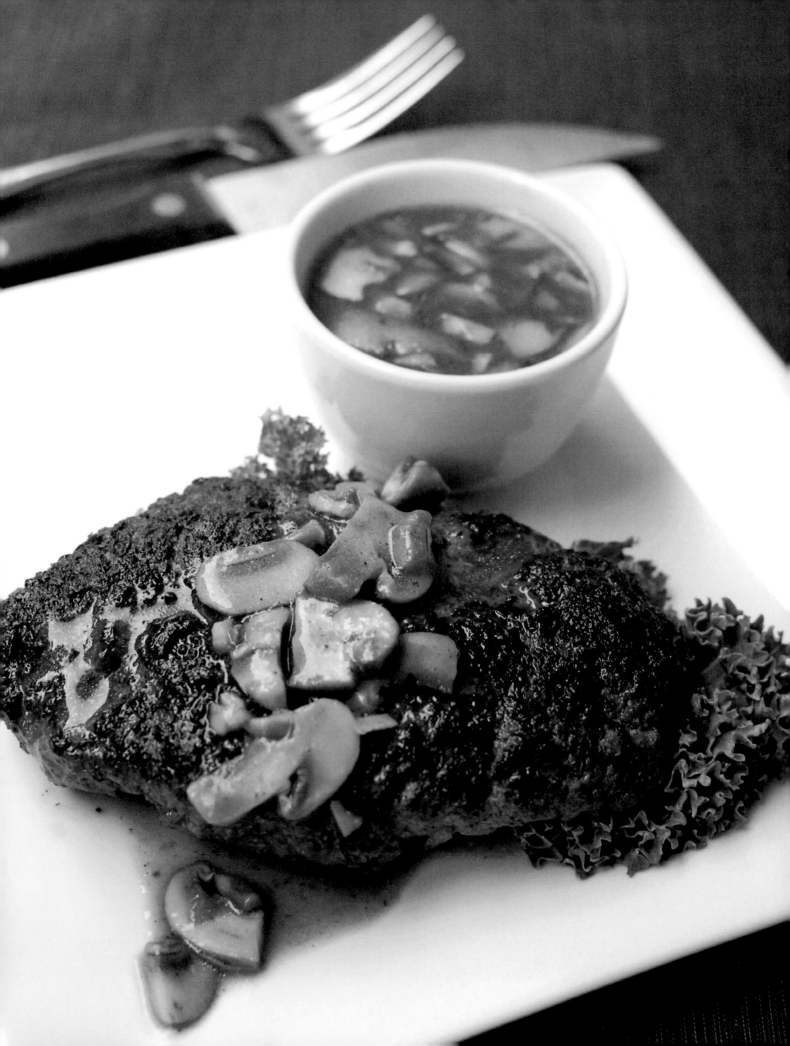

Paleo Pizza Crust

Makes one 9-inch crust
Dairy Free • Fish Free

Yeast Mixture

¼ cup (60 mL) warm water

2 tsp raw honey

2 tsp active dry yeast

Dry Ingredients

¾ cup (90 g) almond flour

3 TBSP coconut flour, sifted

²/₃ cup (80 g) arrowroot starch

Pinch sea salt

Wet Ingredients

1 egg

2 tsp olive oil

1 tsp raw apple cider vinegar

I've tried the half-dozen or so Paleo pizza crust recipes floating around the Web, but all I could taste was almonds. But with the delicate balance of almond flour and coconut flour in this recipe, you won't feel like you just ate a handful of nuts instead of pizza. Plus, the yeast really gives it the authentic flavor of the real thing. So the next time you're tempted to head to the nearest pizza parlor, try this and satisfy your craving without falling off the Paleo wagon!

1. Preheat the oven to 425°F.

2. Place the yeast ingredients in a small bowl and mix. Let sit about 4-5 minutes to activate and become foamy.

3. Meanwhile, place the dry ingredients in a medium bowl and whisk to combine.

4. Add the yeast and the wet ingredients to the dry ingredients. Mix well with a hand mixer.

5. Scoop mixture onto a parchment-lined baking sheet, using a rubber spatula to spread evenly in a circle.

6. Bake 9-10 minutes. Remove from the oven, carefully flip crust over with a spatula, top with sauce and your favorite toppings, then bake 5-10 minutes more, or until toppings are hot. Slice and enjoy!

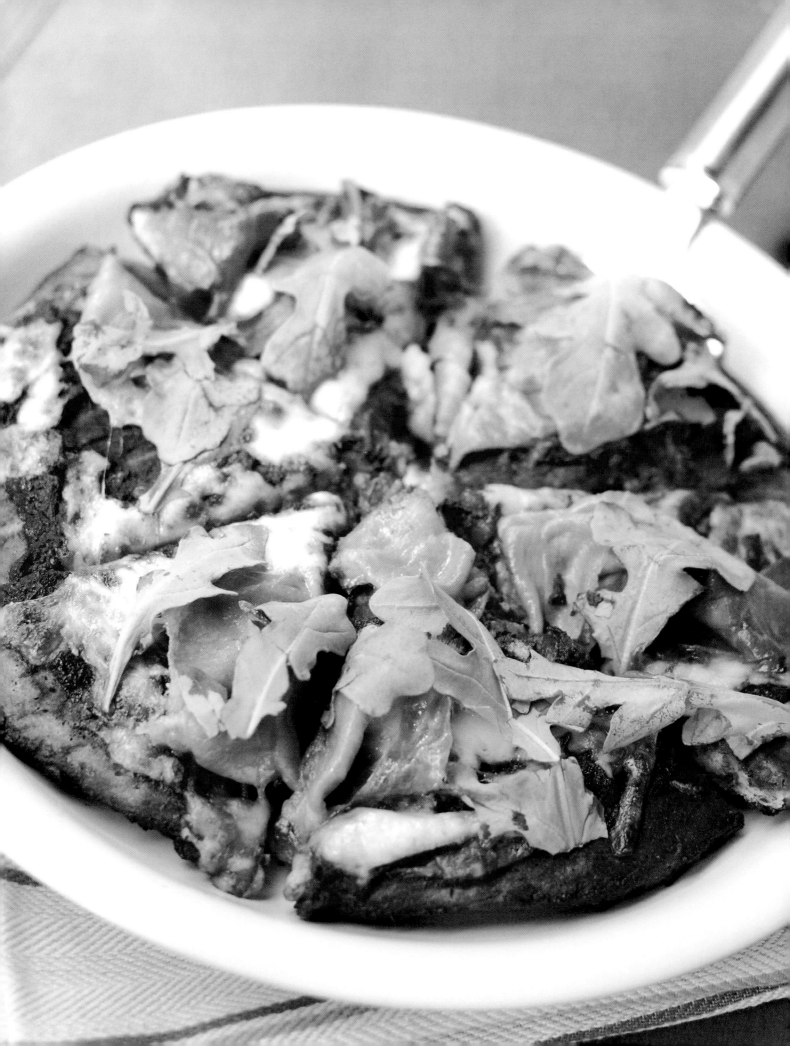

Zucchini Pizza Boats

Makes 4 servings
Dairy Free • Egg Free • Fish Free • Nut Free

Sauce

¼ cup (60 mL) olive oil

1 small onion, diced

1 clove garlic, minced

¼ cup (40 g) chopped parsley

1 28-oz (831 mL) can tomato sauce

2 4-oz (113 g) cans tomato paste

1 28-oz (831 mL) can diced tomatoes

½ tsp oregano

½ tsp basil

Pinch rosemary

1 tsp sea salt

Freshly ground black pepper to taste

Zucchini

4 large zucchini, washed, ends trimmed off, cut in half lengthwise

Toppings of choice (cheese, uncured pepperoni, salami, Italian sausage, ground beef, caramelized onions, black olives, sundried tomatoes, etc.)

We love pizza now and again, but honestly, after going Paleo, crusts, even Paleo versions, aren't something we want or need all the time. And what's a crust anyway, but a topping holder? These zucchini boats answer the call for pizza flavor—they're all topping, no wasted carbs. Not to mention that kids devour the veggies without even realizing it! Score one for Mom!

1. Preheat the oven to 400°F.

2. Heat the oil in a large pot over medium heat. Add the onion and cook until soft, about 5 minutes.

3. Add the garlic and parsley. Stir.

4. Add the remaining sauce ingredients, stirring well to combine. Turn the heat down to low and simmer, covered, for 30 minutes.

5. Meanwhile, clean and prep the zucchini. With a spoon, hollow out the middle of each half, removing only enough flesh to make a shallow well. Place the zucchini on a parchment-lined baking sheet, hollowed-out side up.

6. Spoon some sauce into each zucchini. Top with your favorite items.

7. Bake about 20 minutes, or until toppings are cooked, sauce is bubbling, and zucchini are soft.

Note:
To make a true pizza sauce, I like to purée mine with an immersion blender. Store leftover sauce in small Mason jars in the freezer.

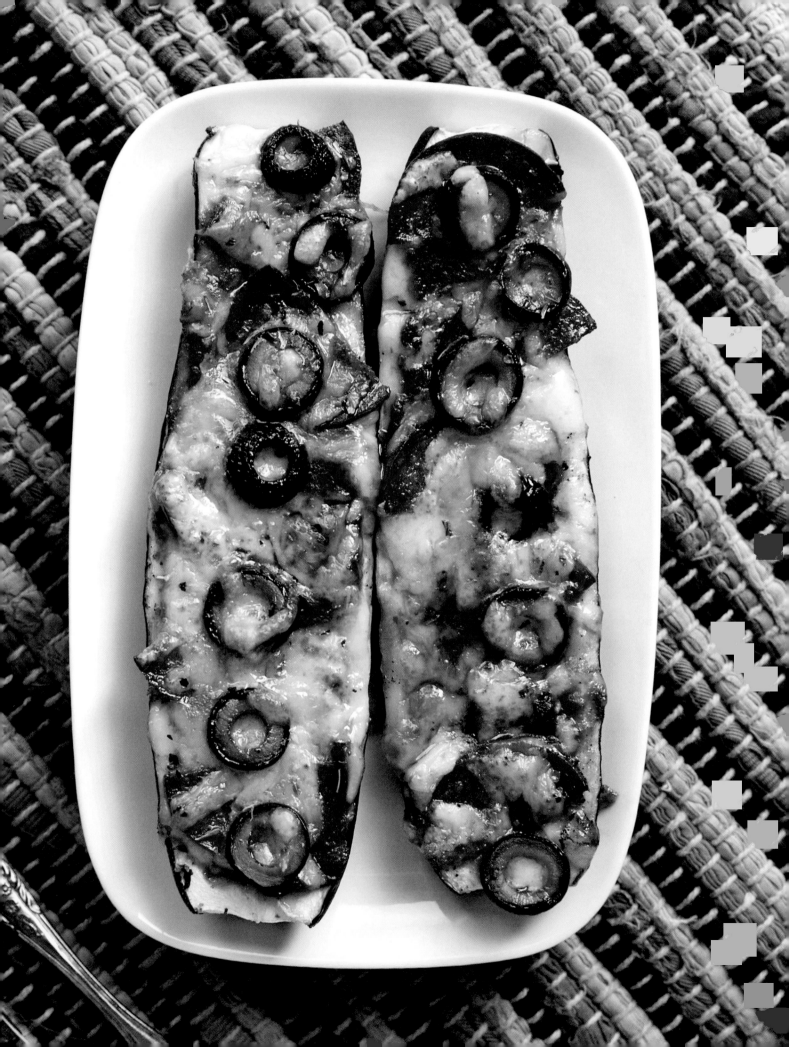

Chinese Pepper Steak

Makes 4 servings

Dairy Free • Egg Free • Fish Free • Nut Free

2 TBSP coconut oil

1 lb (450 g) minute steaks, or round steak, cut into strips (US Wellness Meats)

½ cup (75 g) chopped onion

1 clove garlic, minced

1½ cups (225 g) sliced mushrooms

1 cup (150 g) sliced green or red bell peppers

½ tsp Chinese 5 spice powder

1 tsp freshly grated ginger

½ cup (120 mL) chicken or beef broth, preferably homemade

2 TBSP coconut aminos

This recipe is great for weekdays because in just a few minutes, you can be eating a warm, satisfying, super tasty dinner without breaking a sweat. My favorite kind of meal! We like this one as is, but try serving it over mashed sweet potatoes, cooked spaghetti squash, or cauliflower rice.

1. Heat the oil over medium-high heat in a large skillet. Add the meat and sauté until browned, about 1 minute.

2. Stir in the onions, garlic, mushrooms, and peppers. Cook until tender, about 12 minutes.

3. Sprinkle in the 5 spice and ginger. Add the stock and aminos; stir well.

4. Bring to a boil. Turn heat to medium and simmer, uncovered, about 3-4 minutes, or until sauce has thickened a bit.

5. Serve!

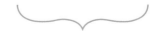

Note:

If you like an even thicker sauce, combine the stock, aminos, and 2 teaspoons arrowroot starch in a bowl before adding to the pan. Simmer 1-2 minutes until sauce thickens.

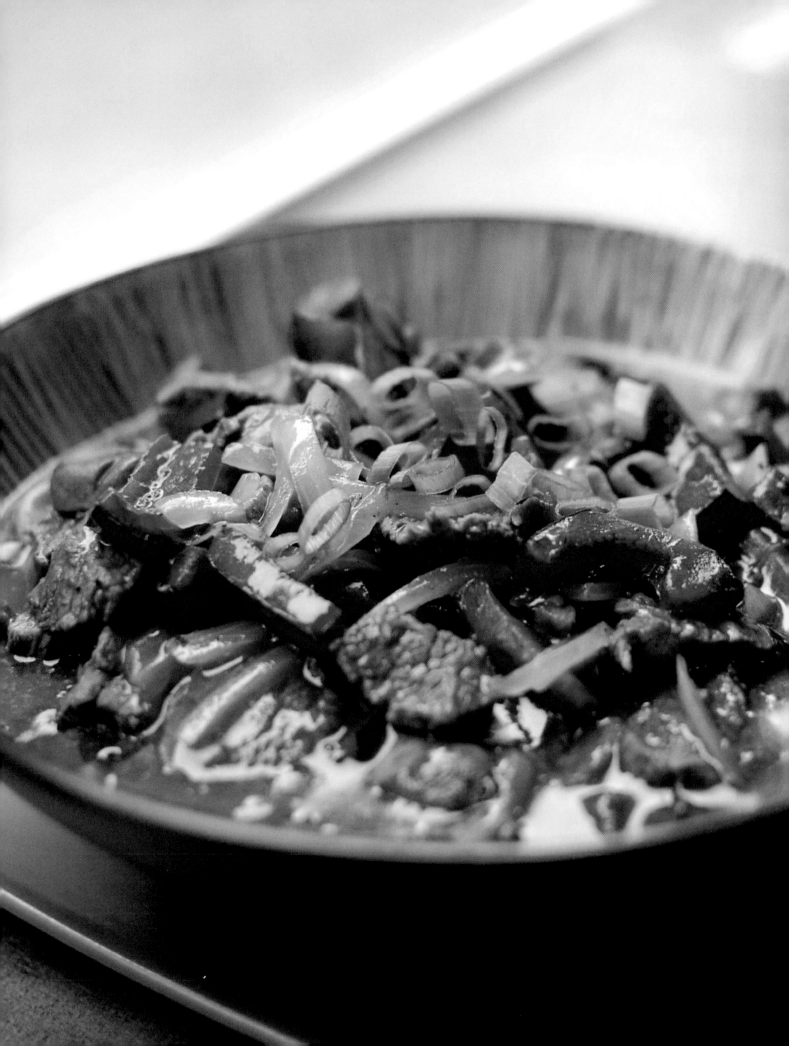

Mandarin Chicken

Makes 4 servings

Dairy Free • Egg Free • Fish Free • Nut Free

Sauce

½ cup (120 mL) frozen orange juice concentrate, thawed

Zest of 1 orange

2 TBSP coconut aminos

1 TBSP walnut or olive oil

2 garlic cloves, minced

1 TBSP raw honey

¼ tsp red chili pepper flakes

Chicken

1 TBSP coconut oil

2 lbs (900 g) boneless, skinless chicken thighs, cut into bite-size pieces (US Wellness Meats)

Sea salt and freshly ground black pepper to taste

½ tsp granulated onion

Add Ons

Diced green onions

Sesame seeds

Many times in a pinch, a long, long time ago, we would buy the frozen Mandarin chicken at our local Trader Joe's. It was tasty and convenient, but while it didn't contain the artificial ingredients and MSG most frozen foods do, it did contain its fair share of gluten and sugar. After playing with this recipe for a few years, I have finally developed a replacement my kids love and I feel good about serving. The trick here is to use concentrated orange juice, because fresh-squeezed just doesn't deliver the intense flavor needed to make this dish pop!

1. Place the sauce ingredients in a small bowl, mix, and set aside.

2. Heat the oil in a large skillet over medium-high heat.

3. Place the chicken in a medium bowl and season lightly with salt, pepper, and the granulated onion. Add the chicken to the hot skillet. Let it brown on all sides, stirring only occasionally, until almost done, about 5 minutes.

4. Add the sauce to the skillet, stirring up the yummy bits from the bottom of the pan as it bubbles. Turn the heat to medium and simmer the sauce, uncovered, about 5 more minutes, or until sauce has thickened a bit and really sticks to the chicken. Serve and enjoy!

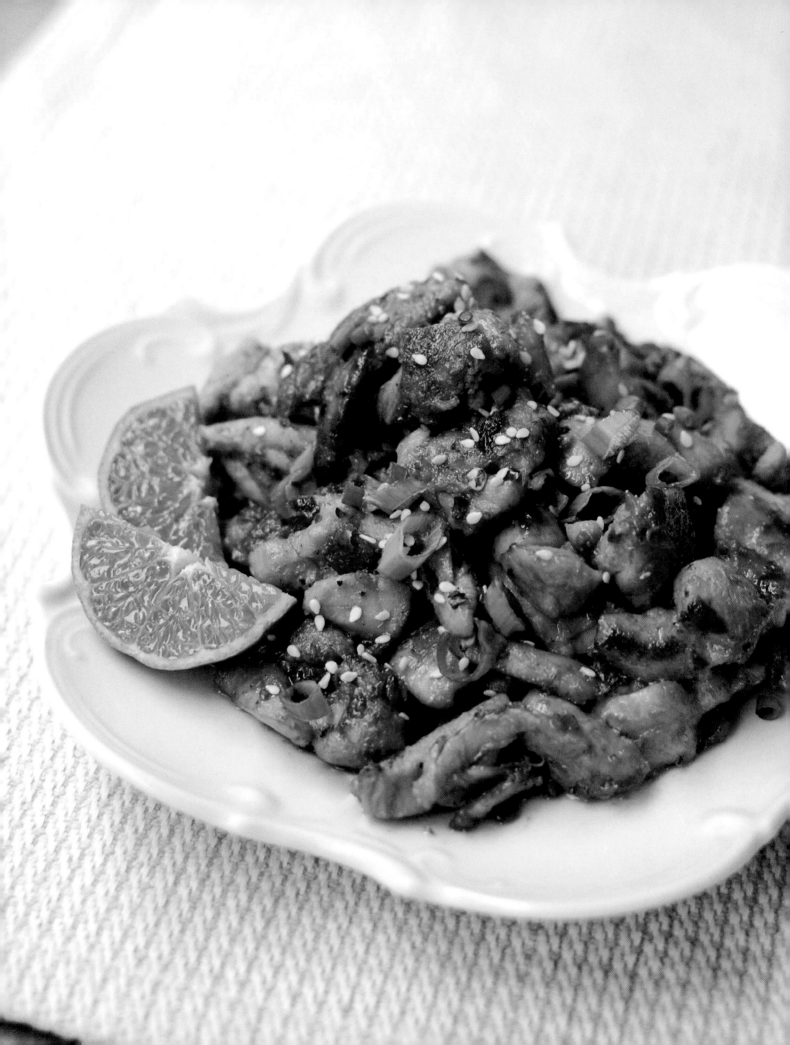

Broccoli Beef

Makes 4 servings

Dairy Free • Egg Free • Nut Free

Sauce

⅓ cup (80 mL) coconut aminos

2 TBSP fish sauce (see "Resources")

2 tsp minced fresh ginger

2 garlic cloves, minced

½ cup (120 mL) water

¼ cup (60 mL) raw honey or pure maple syrup

2 TBSP arrowroot starch

Broccoli

2 tsp coconut oil

4 cups (600 g) broccoli florets

Beef

1 TBSP coconut oil

1 lb (450 g) flank steak, skirt steak, or minute steak, cut into thin strips (US Wellness Meats)

Restaurant broccoli beef is typically coated in cornstarch and fried until slightly crispy—not the best way to keep our Paleo-esque figures. My take delivers on the traditional flavors without the traditional frying in rancid vegetable oil. And feel free to add any chopped veggies you'd like! We usually add sliced peppers, carrots, and green onions for a beautiful veggie-loaded dish.

1. Place the sauce ingredients in a small bowl, mix, and set aside.

2. Cook the broccoli: Heat the coconut oil over high heat in a wok or large skillet. Stir-fry the broccoli 5 minutes. Remove from the wok.

3. Cook the meat: Heat the coconut oil in the wok and stir-fry the meat until almost done, about 4 minutes.

4. Add the broccoli and the sauce to the wok with the meat. Heat until boiling. Continue cooking until the sauce is thickened slightly, about 2-3 minutes.

5. Serve as-is or over cauliflower rice or cooked spaghetti squash!

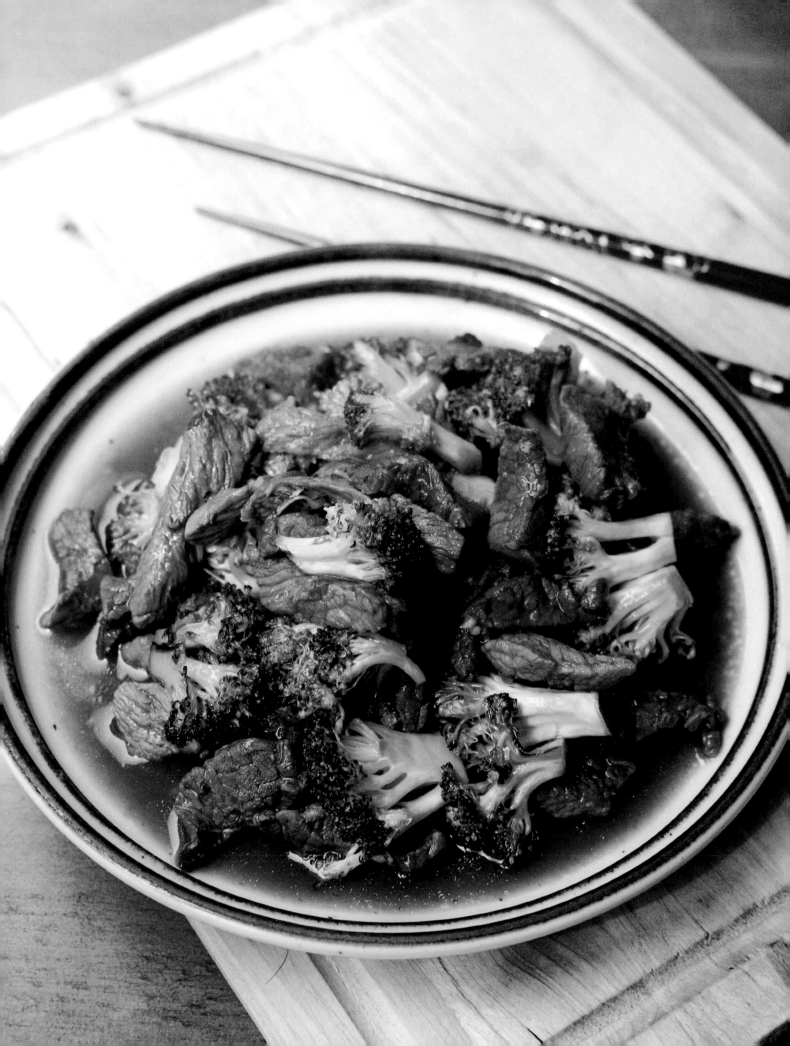

Asian Pork Lettuce Cups

Makes 4 servings
Dairy Free • Egg Free • Nut Free*

Sauce

⅓ cup (80 mL) coconut aminos

2 TBSP fish sauce (see "Resources")

⅓ cup (80 mL) raw apple cider vinegar

Filling

2 TBSP coconut oil

1 lb (450 g) ground pork or boneless pork chops, sliced into bite-size pieces (US Wellness Meats)

8 oz (230 g) white mushrooms, chopped

1 tsp freshly grated ginger

2 garlic cloves, minced

Add Ons

1 head romaine or butter lettuce, washed, leaves separated

Diced carrots

Diced green onions

Diced cucumber

Sesame seeds

Toasted almonds (*optional)

These remind me of those chicken lettuce wraps at many Asian restaurants. Of course, with much better ingredients! The best part is, you can play with the recipe and use anything from ground beef to diced chicken and still get great results. Feel free to add a little heat with some red chili flakes!

1. Place the sauce ingredients in a small bowl, mix, and set aside.

2. Heat the oil in a large skillet over medium-high heat. Add the pork. Cook about 1 minute, stirring occasionally.

3. Add the mushrooms, ginger, and garlic. Cook about 4 minutes, stirring occasionally, or until some of the liquid has evaporated.

4. Stir in the sauce. Bring to a boil. Turn the heat to low and simmer 4-5 minutes, or until the pork is cooked through.

5. To serve, cup a lettuce leaf in your hand, spoon some pork mixture into it, and top with your favorite garnishes.

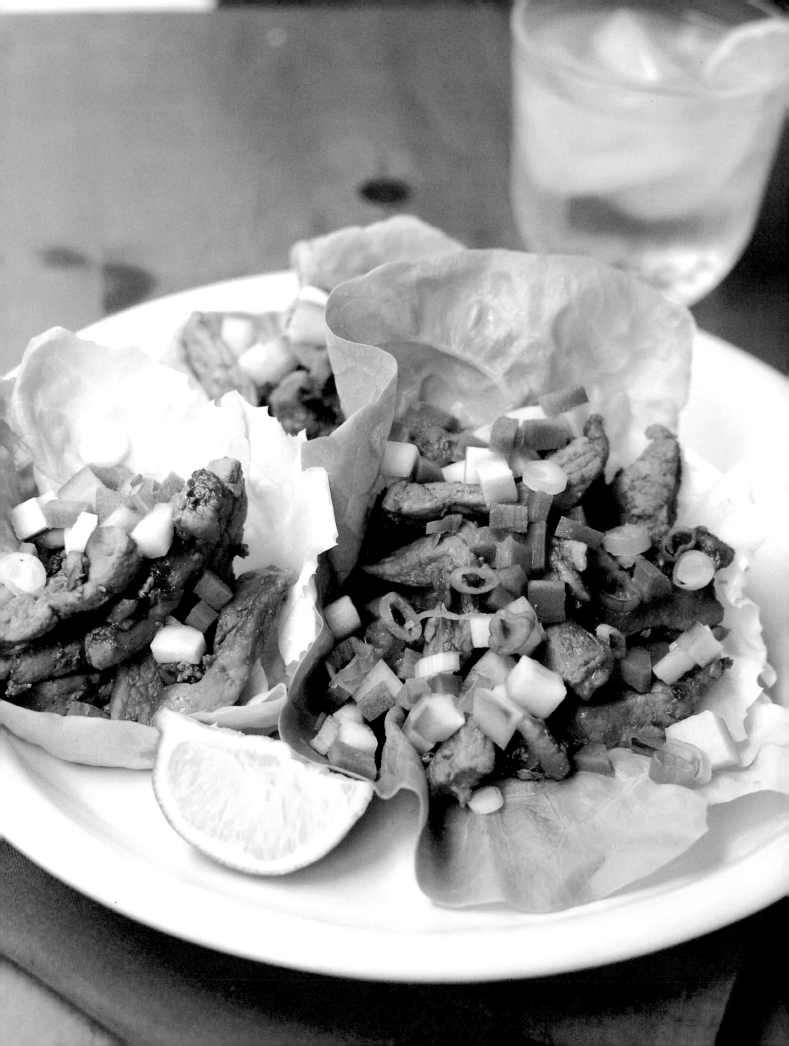

Taro Soft Tacos

Makes 4 to 6 servings

Dairy Free • Egg Free • Fish Free • Nut Free

Shells

About ½ cup (120 mL) coconut oil

1 large taro root, about 3 lbs (1,350 g), sliced into thin discs. (It's best to use a mandoline, so the slices are thin and consistent and thus cook evenly.)

Sea salt

Meat

2 lbs (900 g) ground beef (US Wellness Meats)

2 TBSP Taco Seasoning (recipe follows)

¼ cup (60 mL) water

Shmear

Flesh of 1 avocado, mashed

Sea salt and freshly ground black pepper

Pinch granulated onion

Add Ons

Shredded lettuce

Diced tomatoes

Diced avocado

Sliced black olives

Salsa

If you haven't tried taro yet, I highly recommend it for an occasional, starchy indulgence. Taro is a root veggie native to Southeast Asia and is believed to be one of the earliest cultivated plants. We order the roots from our local Whole Foods and turn them into chips or these soft taco shells. The thinly sliced root crisps up nicely when cooked in coconut oil, but then softens once you load it up with your favorite fillings. Taro adds just the right amount of chew for that soft taco or burrito experience, without gluten or grains or the accompanying bloat.

1. Make the shells: Heat the oil over medium-high heat in a nonstick skillet. Cook the taro until browned on both sides. Remove to a plate and sprinkle lightly with sea salt.

2. Cook the beef: In a large skillet over medium heat, sauté the beef until no longer pink.

3. Sprinkle the taco seasoning over the meat. Add the water and stir. Simmer on low, uncovered, 5 minutes.

4. Meanwhile, make your avocado shmear: Place the avocado in a bowl. Season to taste with a little sea salt, pepper, and granulated onion. Stir to combine.

5. Spread the taro shells with avocado shmear. Spoon some beef on top. Top with your favorite garnishes. Enjoy!

Taco Seasoning:

2 TBSP chili powder

1½ TBSP paprika

1 TBSP cumin

1 TBSP granulated onion

2½ tsp granulated garlic

1 TBSP sea salt

Pinch cayenne

1. Place all the ingredients in a small bowl and mix to combine. Store in an airtight jar. Use 1½ tablespoons to replace 1 packet store-bought taco seasoning, good for 1 pound ground beef.

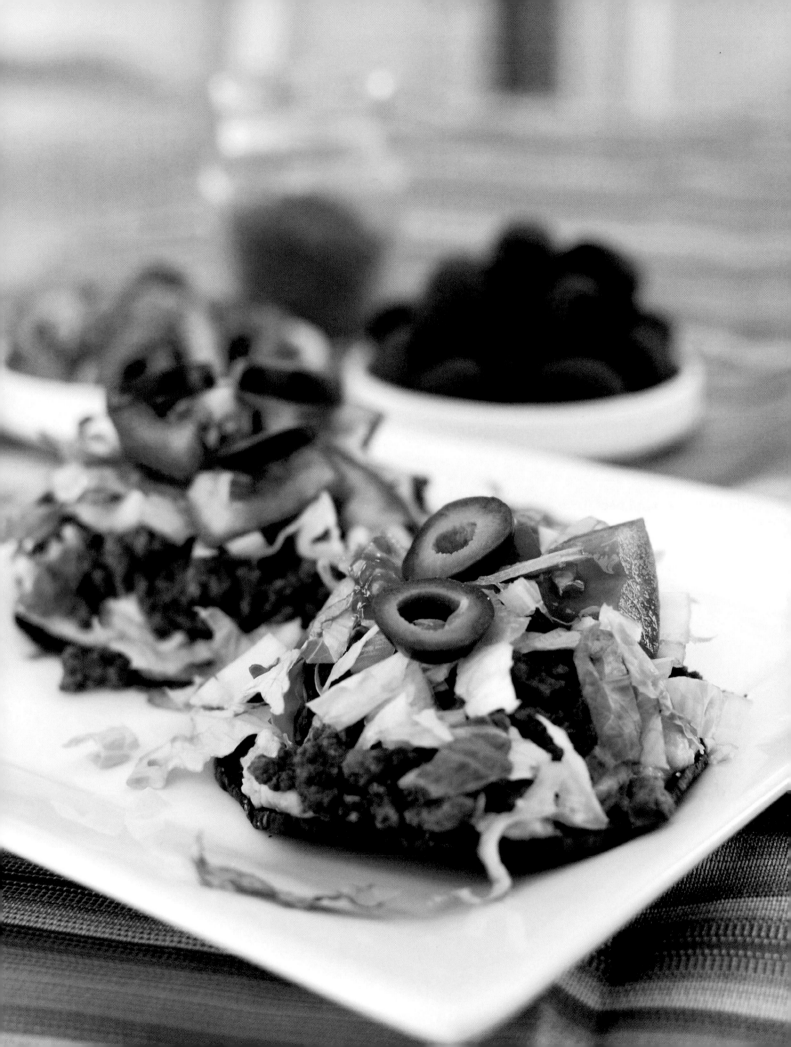

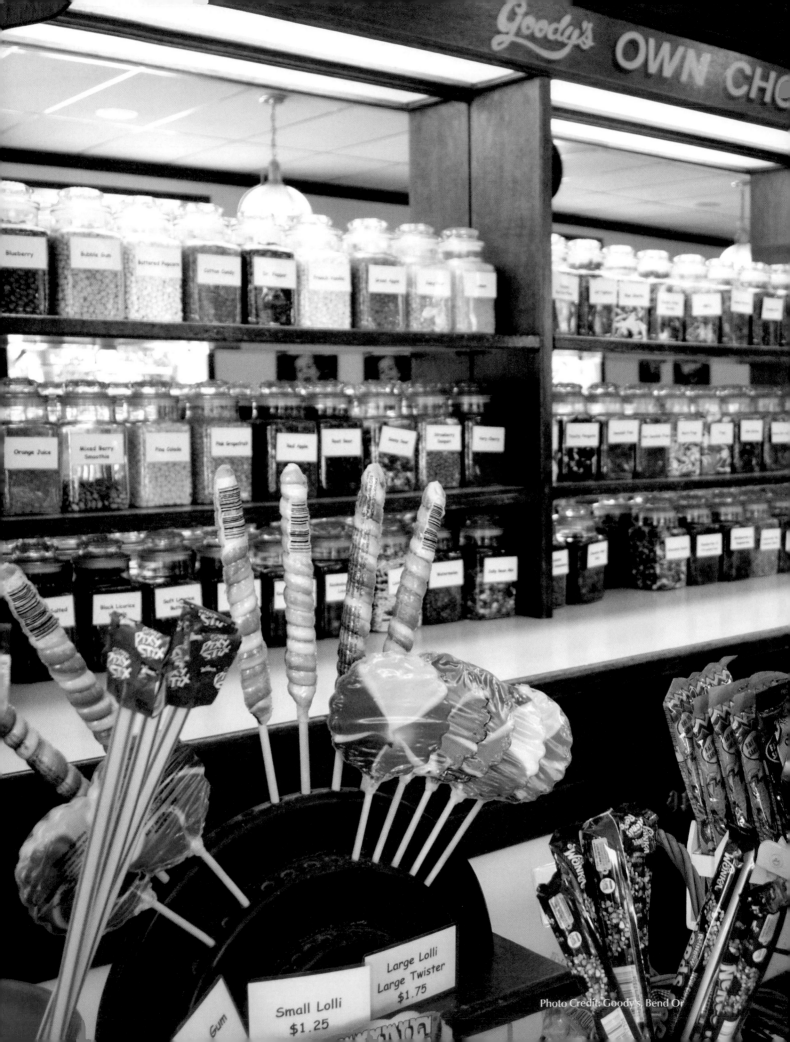

Goody's OWN CHO

Large Lolli
Large Twister
$1.75

Small Lolli
$1.25

The Candy Counter

Almond o' Joys!

Makes about 30 pieces
Dairy Free • Egg Free • Fish Free

Bars

2 cups (180 g) unsweetened finely shredded coconut

⅓ cup (80 mL) raw honey (softened if necessary)

½ cup (60 g) almond flour (Bob's Red Mill is o.k.)

¼ cup (60 mL) coconut oil, melted

Pinch sea salt

60 or so whole roasted, salted almonds

Topping

2 oz (56 g) dark chocolate, chopped

1 oz (28 g) unsweetened dark chocolate (100% cacao), chopped

1 tsp palm shortening or coconut oil

You just can't beat the combination of almonds, coconut, and chocolate. What isn't hard to beat is the stringy, overly sugared coconut that is often a part of that mix. Good-quality, unsweetened coconut provides rich cononutty flavor along with some medium-chain fatty acids and fiber. And you don't have to overdo the chocolate for complete gratification: drizzling the chocolate over the top instead of dunking each bar yields just the right amount of chocolaty taste with a minimum of sugar—just enough to curb your craving without the guilt!

1. Place all the bar ingredients, except the almonds, in a medium bowl and mix until fully combined.

2. Grease an 8-by-8-inch glass baking dish with coconut oil. Press the mixture into the dish. Tip: Wet your hands or place parchment paper or plastic wrap over the mixture to keep it from sticking to your hands.

3. Place the whole almonds in 6 rows over the mixture, and press them in slightly. I place them so that I will have two almonds per piece after they are cut.

4. Place in the freezer until firm, about 15 minutes.

5. Cut into small bars or bite-size cubes. Return to the freezer for 1 hour.

6. Meanwhile, melt the topping ingredients in the top of a double boiler over simmering water and stir until melted.

7. Remove the bars from the baking dish with a spatula and space them evenly on a parchment-lined baking sheet. Drizzle melted chocolate over the tops of each.

8. Place the bars in the refrigerator until chocolate is set, about 30 minutes. Store in an airtight container in the fridge up to 1 week, or in the freezer up to 3 months.

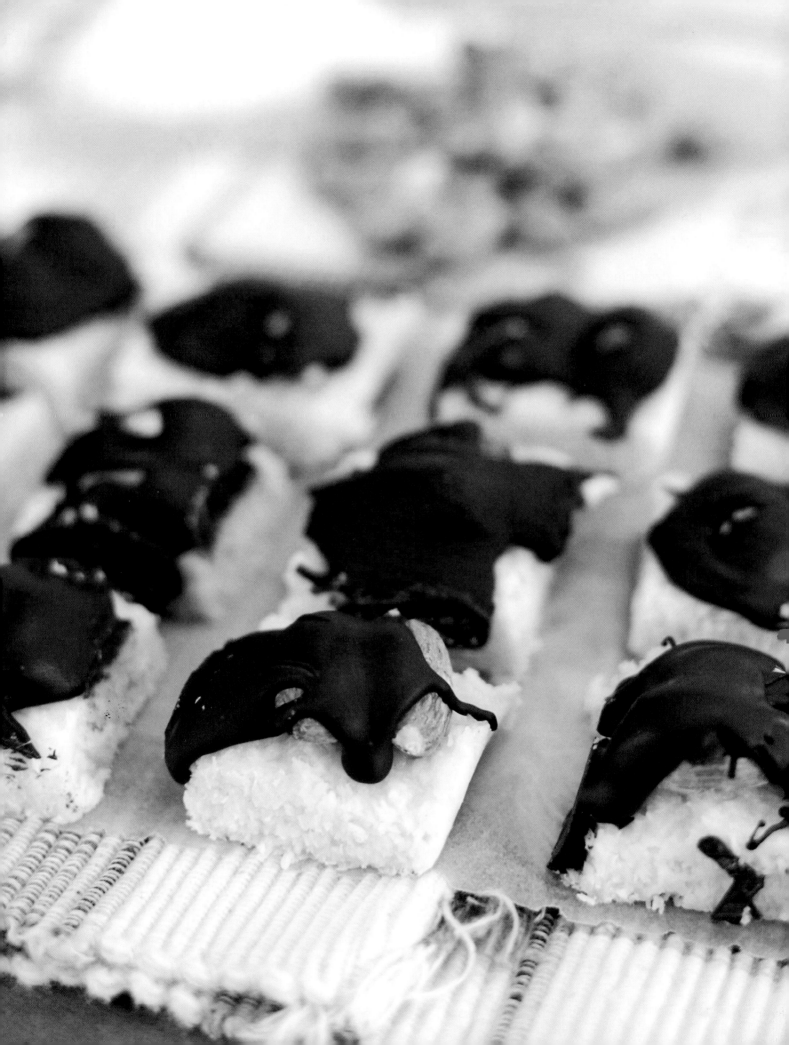

Peppermint Creams

Makes about 10 patties
Dairy Free • Egg Free • Fish Free • Nut Free

Creams

⅓ cup (80 mL) pure maple syrup (cold)

2 tsp coconut flour, sifted

½ tsp pure vanilla extract

½ tsp pure peppermint extract (or a little more for more intense flavor)

2 TBSP coconut butter, softened

Pinch sea salt

½ cup (120 mL) coconut oil, melted

Coating

½ cup (80 g) chopped dark chocolate

2 oz (56 g) unsweetened dark chocolate (100% cacao), chopped

¼ tsp pure peppermint extract

If you've ever tried to make peppermint creams with coconut oil and then spent an hour cursing as the temperature-sensitive oil melted the chocolate coating off as soon as you dipped it, you will greatly appreciate this recipe. Dark chocolate hugs the creamy, minty, sturdy center and doesn't let go, thanks to the addition of coconut butter. You'll never miss the sugar-laden originals with these decadent bites around!

1. Make the creams: Place all the ingredients, except the coconut oil, in a small bowl and use a hand mixer to combine.

2. With the mixer on low, slowly pour in the coconut oil. Mix until fully incorporated.

3. Chill the mixture until firm, about 1 hour.

4. Scoop the mixture into small balls, then press them between the palms of your hands to form patties.

5. Freeze the patties on a parchment-lined baking sheet until hard.

6. Make the coating: Melt the topping ingredients in the top of a double boiler over simmering water and stir until melted. Cool for 5 minutes.

7. Using 2 forks, dip the frozen patties in the chocolate, scraping off the excess on the side of the bowl. Place on the parchment-lined baking sheet.

8. Freeze until chocolate hardens. Store in an airtight container in the fridge up to 1 week, or in the freezer up to 3 months.

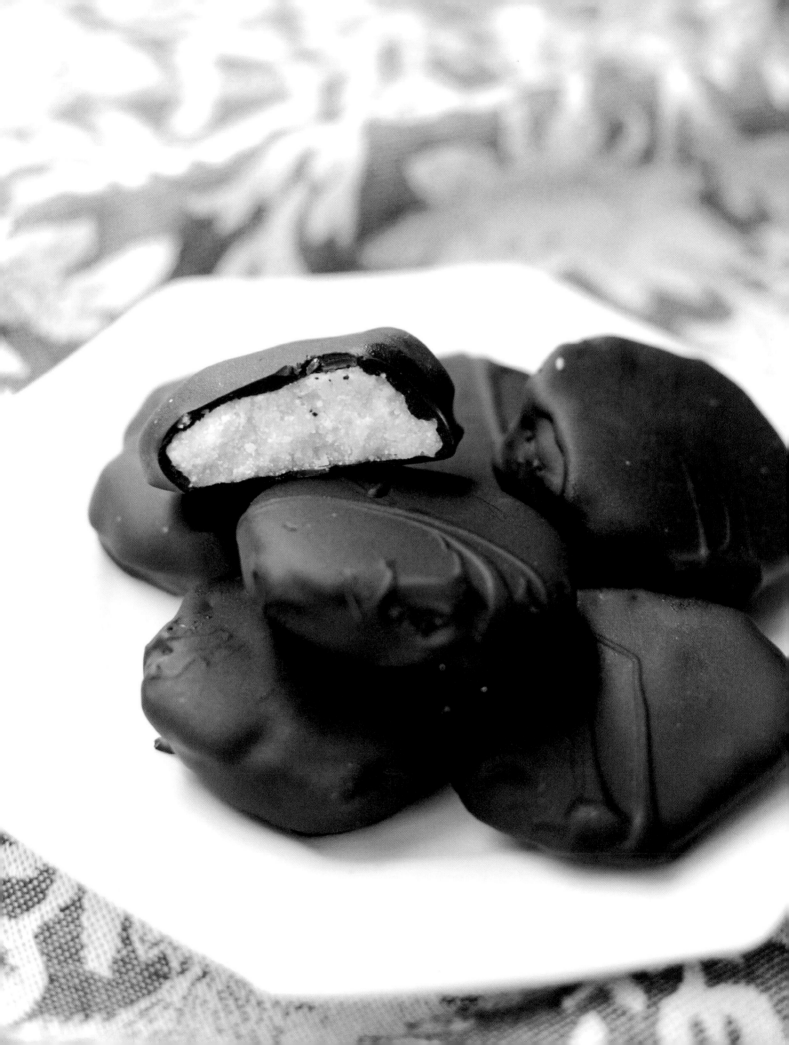

Sun Butter Bark

Makes about 2 cups

Dairy Free • Egg Free • Fish Free • Nut Free

1 cup (240 mL) coconut oil, softened

¼ cup (60 g) sugar-free sunflower seed butter

2 tsp pure maple syrup

½ tsp pure vanilla extract

Pinch sea salt

1 oz (28 g) dark chocolate, chopped fine

This is my all-time favorite coconut bark! I guess it reminds me of the classic peanut butter–chocolate combo, except now I can enjoy it guilt, and stomach-ache, free! Go wild and experiment by using your favorite nut butter. My youngest cannot tolerate nuts, so she was thrilled to have this little treat made especially for her!

1. Place all the ingredients, except the chocolate, in a medium bowl and mix to combine.

2. Pour onto a parchment-lined baking sheet.

3. Sprinkle with chopped chocolate.

4. Place the baking sheet in the freezer for at least 30 minutes, or until bark is hard.

5. Break into pieces and enjoy! Store in an airtight container in the freezer up to 1 month.

Note:

Coconut oil is solid at temperatures under 76°F and liquid above. So if you're making this in the summer months and your oil is liquefied, simply place the oil in the fridge until it firms up, then, let it sit out until it's the consistency of really soft butter. If your oil is solid, simply microwave for a few seconds at a time, stirring in between, until it's soft. You still want it to be white, not clear.

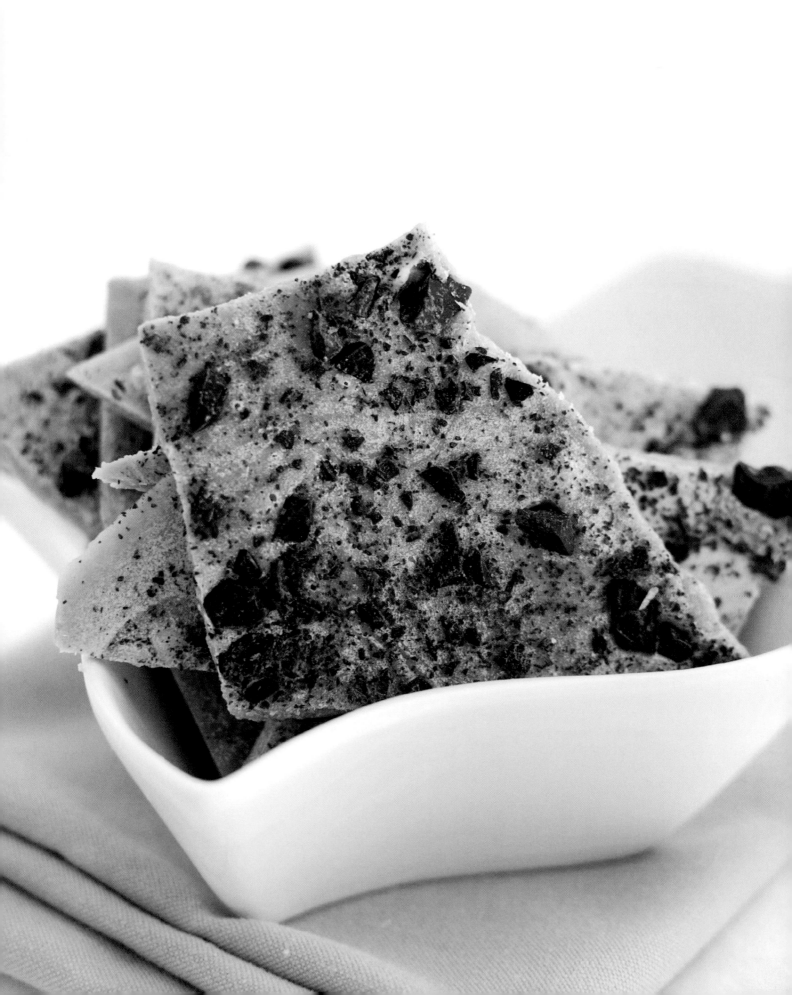

Chocolate-Cherry Coconut Bark

Makes about 2 cups
Dairy Free • Egg Free • Fish Free

1 cup (240 mL) coconut oil,
softened

½ tsp pure vanilla extract

⅛ tsp pure almond extract

2 TBSP chopped, dried
unsweetened cherries

1 TBSP mini chocolate chips
or dark chocolate shavings

Pinch sea salt

Few drops beet juice for
color (see Note)

Sometimes, small things make a big visual impact. For this decadent coconut bark, the pink color really makes it taste better. Really! At least that's what my kids tell me. Coconut oil + cherries + dark chocolate + beet juice = one nutritional stud-muffin of a mouth-watering snack. My kiddos love to munch on it after school, and with a snack this healthy, I have no reason to say no!

1. Place all ingredients in a medium bowl and mix to combine.

2. Pour the mixture onto a parchment-lined baking sheet and spread evenly with a spoon.

3. Freeze until hard. Break into pieces and dig in. Store in an airtight container in freezer up to 1 month.

Note:
To make beet juice, peel and slice 1 large beet. Boil in a small saucepan with just enough water to cover the beets, for 10 minutes. Cool for 15 minutes. Strain the beets from the juice and store juice in a small Mason jar. I keep mine in the freezer, then when I need it, I simply defrost it just enough to get a few drops of liquid out, and refreeze. It doesn't take much to add great color to foods, so this should last you awhile.

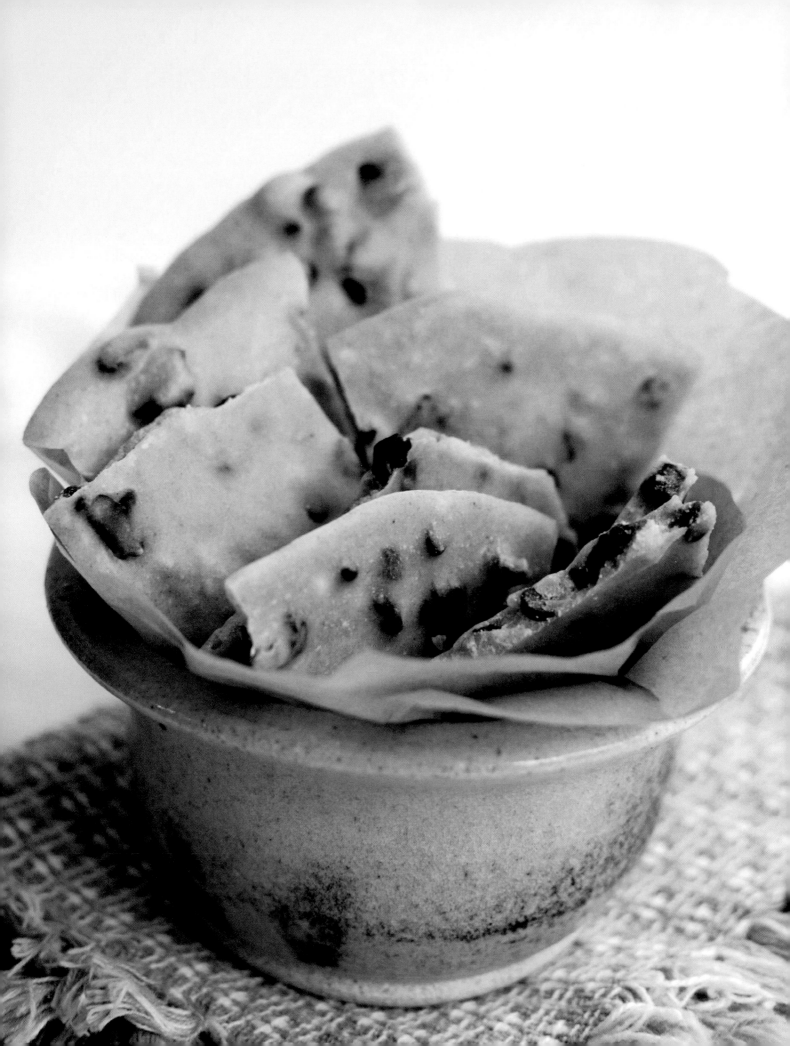

Mint-Chip Coconut Bark

Makes about 2 cups
Dairy Free • Egg Free • Fish Free • Nut Free

1 cup (240 mL) coconut oil, softened

½ tsp pure vanilla extract

½ tsp pure peppermint extract

1-2 TBSP dark chocolate shavings or mini dark chocolate chips (amount depends on how sweet you want it)

Pinch sea salt

Another one of our favorite flavor combinations! Enjoy the cool, refreshing taste of a peppermint patty without all the work or sugar. And the best part is, a small piece is extremely satisfying thanks to the coconut oil, so you will find it difficult to overindulge on this one.

1. Place all ingredients in a medium bowl and mix to combine.

2. Pour the mixture onto a parchment-lined baking sheet and spread evenly with a spoon.

3. Freeze until hard. Break into pieces and enjoy! Store in an airtight container in the freezer up to 1 month.

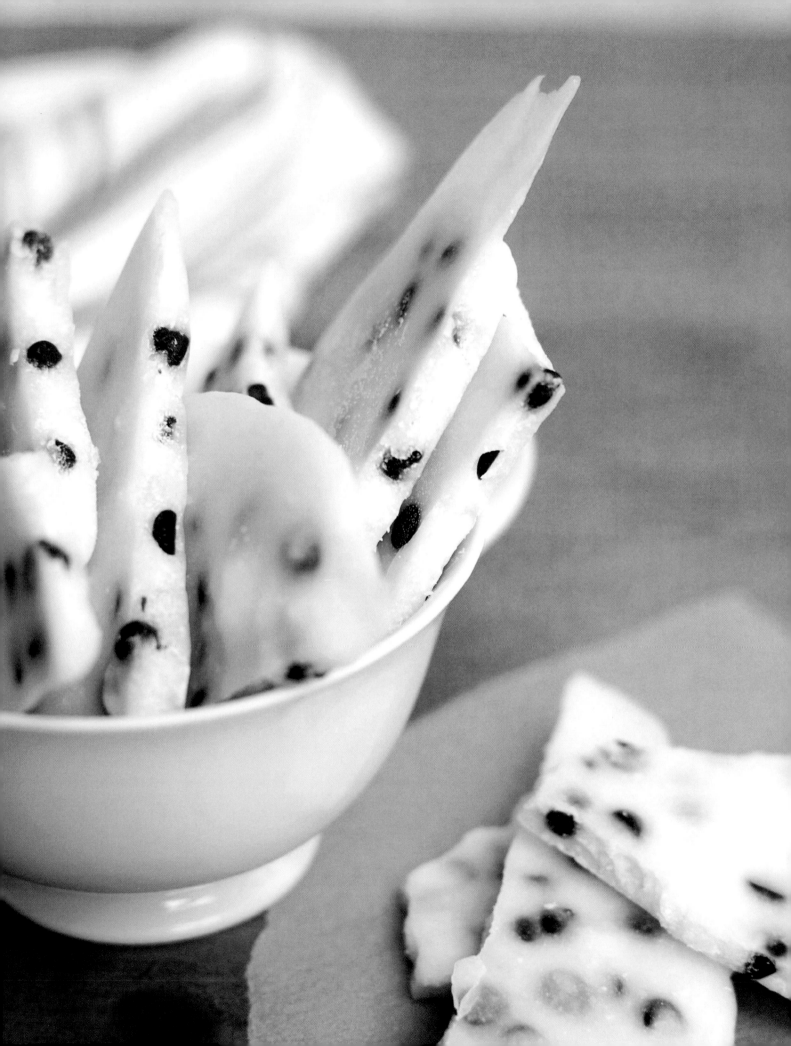

Toffee Caramels

Makes about 24 pieces
Dairy Free • Egg Free • Fish Free

Toffee

1 tsp pure vanilla extract

⅓ cup (80 g) almond butter

¼ cup (50 g) coconut crystals
(palm sugar)

½ cup (120 mL) coconut
nectar

¼ cup (60 mL) water

Coating

⅓ cup (50 g) dark chocolate

1 oz (28 g) unsweetened
dark chocolate (100% cacao),
chopped

1 tsp palm shortening

With a wonderful toffee crunch that turns into a chewy, caramel-like candy, you'll think you're eating the real thing, but—surprise!—these are dairy-free. Keep in mind that a true toffee is generally cooked to about 300°F on a candy thermometer, which works fine for refined sugar but is tough to do without burning when using unrefined, natural sweeteners such as coconut sugar and nectar. That's why you get crunch plus chew. A perfect holiday gift or treat for Valentine's Day! You're welcome.

1. First, have your vanilla and almond butter measured and ready to go. Set aside.

2. Line a baking sheet with parchment paper.

3. Make the toffee: Place the coconut sugar, coconut nectar, and water in a medium saucepan and heat over medium to medium-high heat, stirring occasionally, until it comes to a boil and the coconut sugar has dissolved.

4. Insert a candy thermometer, being careful not to let it touch the bottom or sides of the pan. Continue boiling until the mixture reaches 285°F.

5. Remove the pan from the heat and quickly add the vanilla and almond butter. Stir to combine.

6. Quickly pour the mixture onto the parchment-lined baking sheet, spreading evenly, to about a ½-inch to ¾-inch thickness.

7. Use a sharp, greased knife to score (don't cut all the way through) into bite-size squares. Continue to score along the same lines every few seconds, until you eventually cut all the way through as it cools down a bit.

8. Cool completely on the baking sheet at room temperature, about 2-3 hours.

9. Meanwhile, make the coating: Place all the coating ingredients in the top of a double boiler over low heat and stir until smooth.

10. Using 2 forks, dip each piece of toffee into the chocolate. Tap off any excess chocolate on the side of the bowl and set back on the parchment-lined baking sheet. Cool until chocolate is set, or place in the fridge to speed the cooling process along.

11. Store toffee in an airtight container in the fridge to keep it crisp. Room-temperature toffee is more like a really chewy caramel.

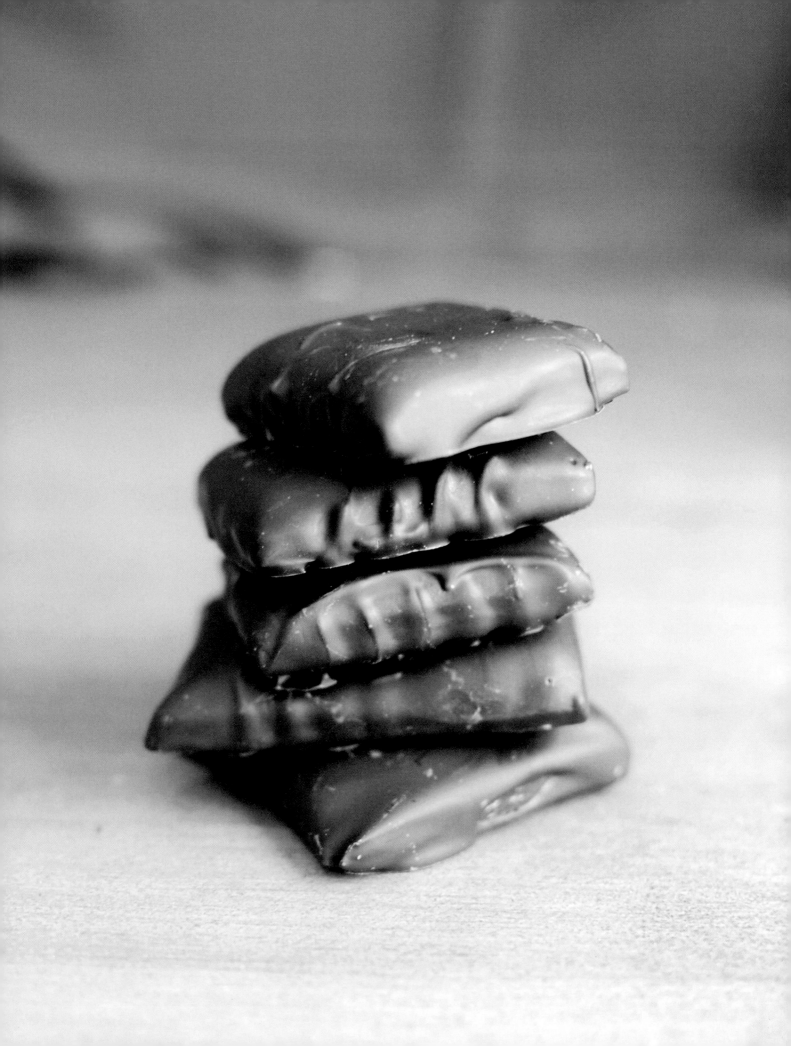

Coconut-Milk Truffles

Makes about 20 truffles
Dairy Free • Egg Free • Fish Free

Truffles

⅓ cup (80 mL) full-fat coconut milk

4 oz (113 g) dark chocolate, chopped

2 oz (56 g) unsweetened dark chocolate (100% cacao), chopped

½ tsp pure vanilla extract

¼ tsp pure almond extract

Toppings

Unsweetened cocoa powder

Finely shredded unsweetened coconut

Finely chopped almonds, pistachios, or macadamias

Ground freeze-dried fruit such as strawberries

Pinch cayenne

Pinch curry powder

A great dairy-free version of the decadent, melt-in-your-mouth truffles from your (once) favorite chocolate boutique. You can get really creative with the toppings, so feel free to improvise! I love the sweet, salty, and slightly spicy combination of sea salt and cayenne. Any way you roll it, you'll be in truffle heaven. And these are so pretty, they make great gifts for Paleo or non-Paleo hostesses.

1. Heat the coconut milk in a medium saucepan over medium heat until it starts to bubble around the edges of the pan. Remove from the heat.

2. Add both chocolates and both extracts. Let mixture sit for a few seconds to allow the chocolate to melt. Whisk until smooth.

3. Place in the refrigerator to cool until firm, about 45 minutes.

4. Use a melon baller to scoop into balls.

5. Roll the balls in desired topping and place in an airtight container. Store in the fridge up to 1 week.

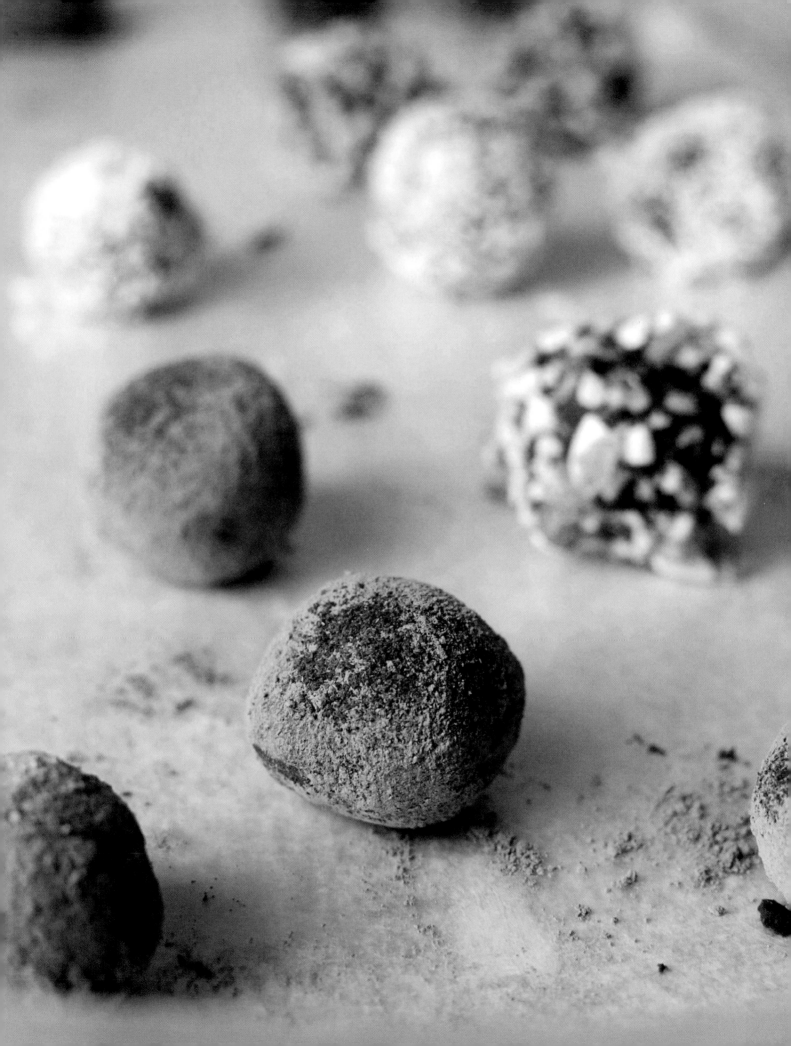

Macadamia-Cherry Clusters

Makes about 10 clusters

Dairy Free • Egg Free • Fish Free

1 cup (160 g) chopped dark chocolate

2 tsp palm shortening

1½ cups (225 g) roasted, salted macadamia nuts

¼ cup (40 g) dried unsweetened cherries

Pinch sea salt

One of my favorite, more frequent indulgences is a small chocolate cluster with a few nuts and a pinch of sea salt. They are so easy to make and so much cheaper than buying them by the pound at the supermarket. Best of all, you get that little hit of something sweet and salty without the chocolate overkill.

1. Place the chocolate and the shortening in the top of a double boiler over gently simmering water and stir occasionally, until almost all the pieces are melted. Remove from the heat and stir until the chocolate is completely melted.

2. Add the macadamias and cherries and stir to combine. The ratio of nuts to chocolate should be high. If the mixture looks too thin, add more nuts.

3. With a tablespoon, scoop clusters and place on a waxed, paper-lined baking sheet.

4. Sprinkle each with a tiny amount of sea salt.

5. Refrigerate until the chocolate is hard. Store in an airtight container up to 2 weeks.

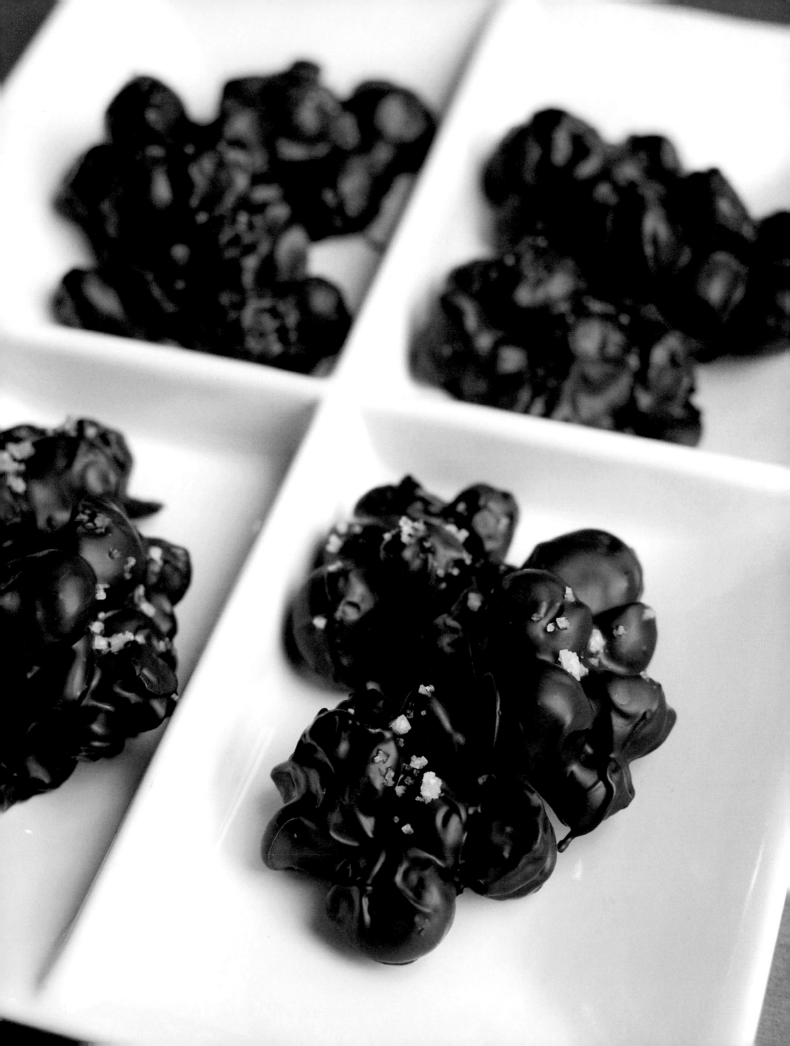

Candied Coconut Walnuts

Makes about 1½ cups
Dairy Free • Egg Free • Fish Free

⅓ cup (80 mL) pure maple syrup

1 cup (150 g) raw walnuts, coarsely chopped

½ cup (45 g) unsweetened coconut flakes

½ tsp pure vanilla extract

Something about the combination of maple, coconut, and walnuts is addicting. This one is hard to stop eating! So make a batch for the kids' lunches, or for a family road trip, and share the addiction to these simple, wholesome ingredients.

1. Preheat the oven to 350°F.

2. Place all ingredients in a small bowl and toss to coat well with syrup.

3. Pour the mixture onto a parchment-lined baking sheet and spread evenly.

4. Bake 15-20 minutes, or until golden brown and bubbling and the coconut flakes are toasted.

5. Cool completely on trays placed on a wire rack.

6. Break into pieces. Store in an airtight container up to 1 week.

Note:
Can't do nuts? Try using raw pumpkin seeds instead!

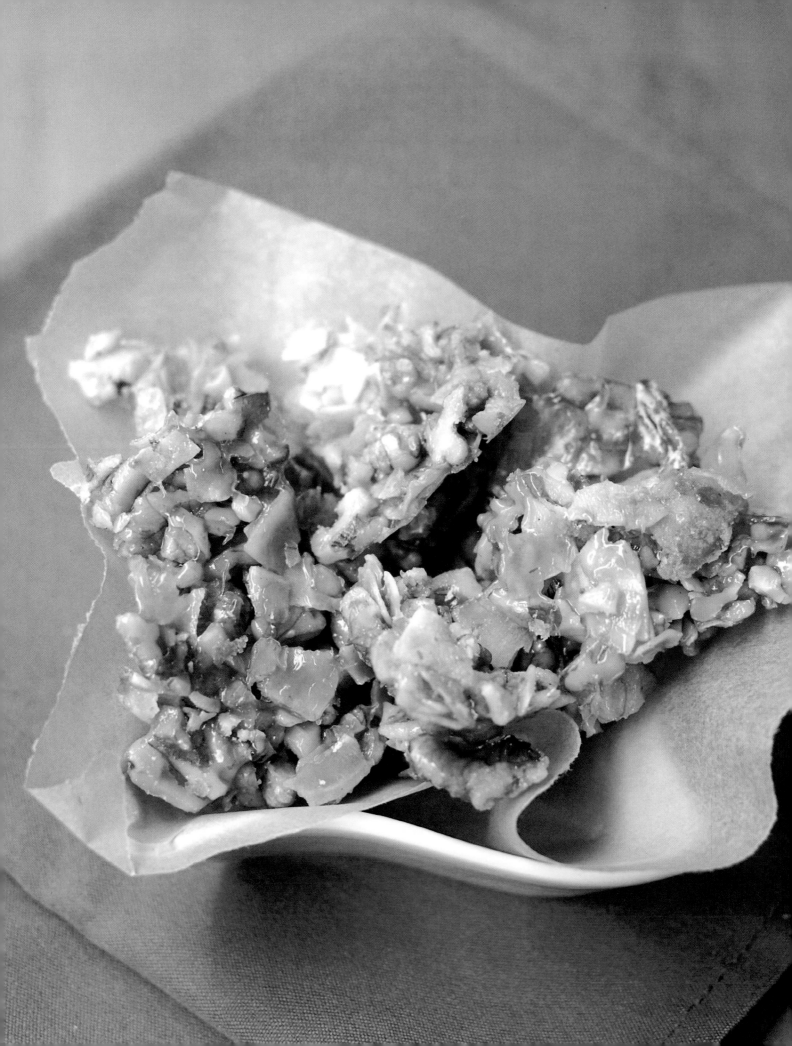

Coconut-Milk Caramels

Makes about 30 pieces
Dairy Free* • Egg Free • Fish Free • Nut Free

Caramel

1 cup (200 g) coconut crystals (palm sugar)

¼ cup (60 mL) coconut nectar

½ cup (120 mL) full-fat coconut milk

⅓ cup (80 g) grass-fed butter (*optional)

Coating

½ cup (80 g) chopped dark chocolate

1 oz (28 g) unsweetened dark chocolate (100% cacao), chopped

This one's for my mom! She was a huge fan of the big 'ol box of Milk Duds at the movie theater as a kid, and she passed that snack habit down to me. Thanks, Mom! Well, weren't we both thrilled to discover these little nuggets of goodness. Chewy, creamy caramel with a touch of sweet, dark chocolate makes a great treat during the holidays, for a gift, or for a movie-night indulgence! Who needs to buy candy with ingredients you can't even pronounce when you can make your own all-natural delights and still stay on the Paleo path?

1. Make the caramel: Place all the caramel ingredients in a medium saucepan and stir to combine.

2. Heat over medium-high heat, and boil mixture until it reaches 250°F on a candy thermometer, about 20 minutes.

3. Remove from the heat and let sit until the caramel is soft and pliable but cool, about 20-30 minutes.

4. Roll the caramel into balls by the teaspoonful and place on a parchment-lined baking sheet.

5. Make the coating: Place all the chocolate in a double boiler over gently simmering water and stir until almost melted. Remove from the heat and stir until completely melted and smooth.

6. With 2 forks, dip each ball of caramel into the chocolate, tapping off any excess on the side of the bowl. Place back on the parchment-lined baking sheet to set. You can refrigerate to speed up the process. Store in an airtight container up to 5 days.

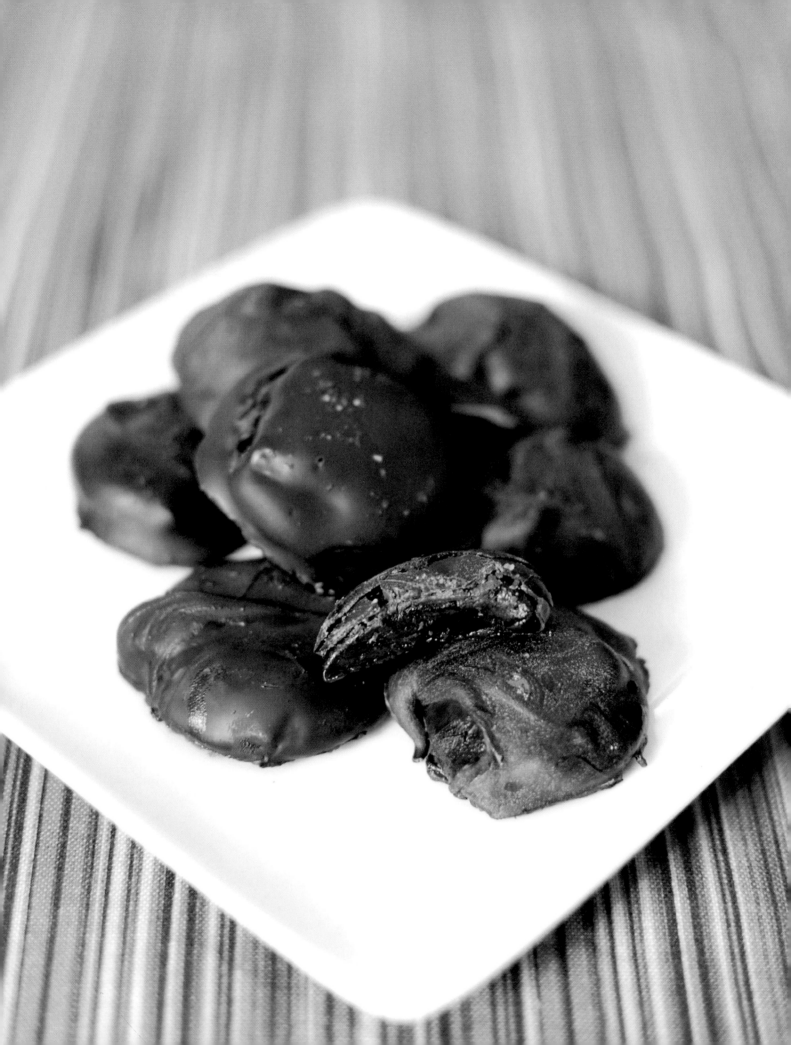

Paleo Marsh-Maleos

Makes about 32 treats

Dairy Free • Egg Free • Fish Free • Nut Free

For Dusting

2 TBSP coconut crystals, powdered (grind in food processor or coffee grinder)

2 TBSP arrowroot starch

Gelatin

½ cup (180 mL) cold water

2 packages unflavored gelatin

Marsh-Maleos

¼ cup (60 mL) water

½ cup (120 mL) raw coconut nectar

½ cup (120 mL) pure maple syrup (or raw honey)

⅛ tsp sea salt

1 TBSP pure vanilla extract

You shouldn't be surprised to find out that I am not a huge fan of marshmallows. They are basically just whipped sugar, high-fructose corn syrup (yuck!), and artificial flavors and colors—not an ounce of nutrition to be found anywhere. But about twice a summer, I am overwhelmed by nostalgia and just have to toast marshmallows over the fire during our family's campout. So what's a Paleo mom to do? Make her own with the best ingredients possible! And, yes, these really do tip the scale when it comes to even natural sweeteners, but at least I am in control of the ingredients and can whip up a safe, rare treat for my kids—and now, so can you!

1. Place the powdered coconut crystals and arrowroot in a small bowl and stir to mix. Set aside. This is your dusting mixture.

2. Lightly grease an 8-by-8-inch glass baking dish with cooking spray, then line it with parchment paper. Spray the parchment with cooking spray and sprinkle enough of the dusting mixture to lightly coat the bottom and sides. (This is easiest with a sifter.) Tap out excess "dust" onto a piece of waxed paper to use later.

3. Make the gelatin: Place ½ cup water in the bowl of a stand mixer fit with a whisk attachment. Sprinkle the gelatin evenly over the water and let sit.

4. Meanwhile, make the Marsh-Maleos: Place the remaining ingredients in a medium saucepan over medium-low heat and stir occasionally until combined.

5. Turn the heat up to medium-high, letting the mixture come to a boil and then simmer until it reaches exactly 240°F on a candy thermometer, about 10 minutes. Immediately remove from heat.

6. Turn mixer on to low. Slowly stream the hot syrup mixture into the gelatin mixture, being very careful not to splash it on yourself! Increase speed to medium and mix for 1 minute.

7. Turn the mixer to high and whip for about 10 minutes, until the mixture is very thick and sticking to the whisk. Like marshmallow cream.

8. Pour the marsh-maleo mixture into the dish. Using a rubber spatula, spread as evenly as possible. Tip: Rinse the spatula often with hot water or spray with cooking spray to prevent sticking.

9. Sprinkle the tops lightly with dusting mixture.

10. Let sit for at least 5 hours at room temperature to firm up.

11. Remove from the pan and cut into squares with a pizza cutter sprayed with cooking spray. Sprinkle each side of each Marsh-Maleo with the dusting mixture to prevent sticking. Store in an airtight container up to 5 days.

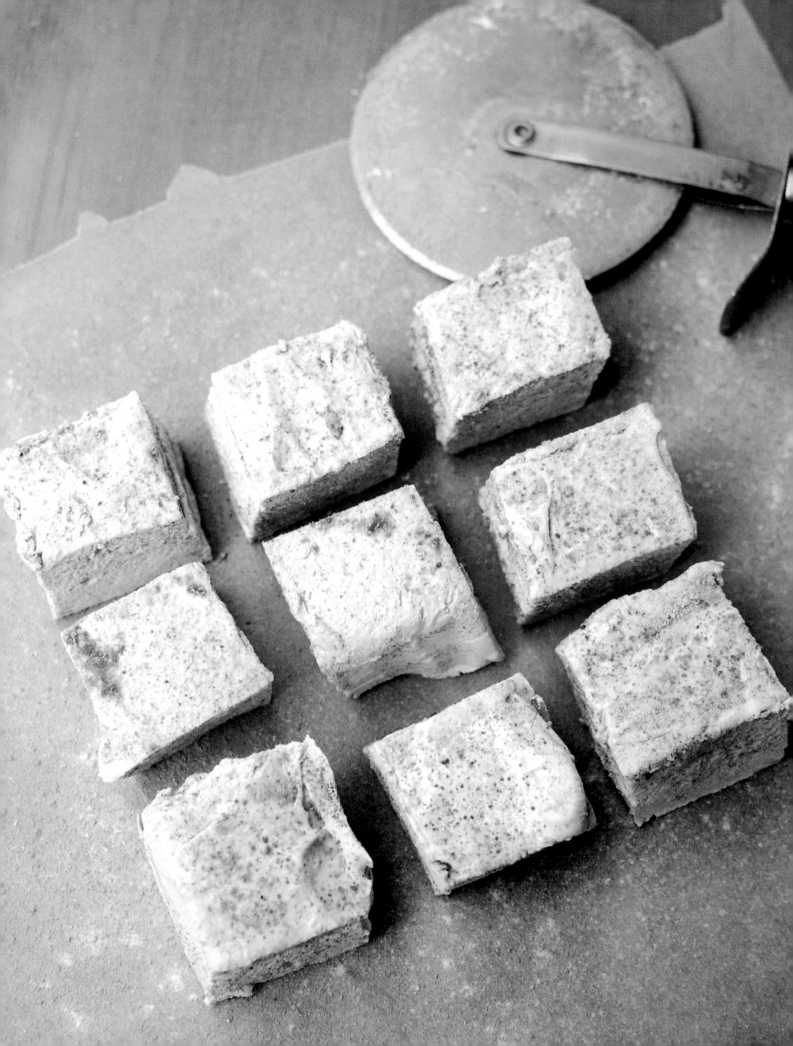

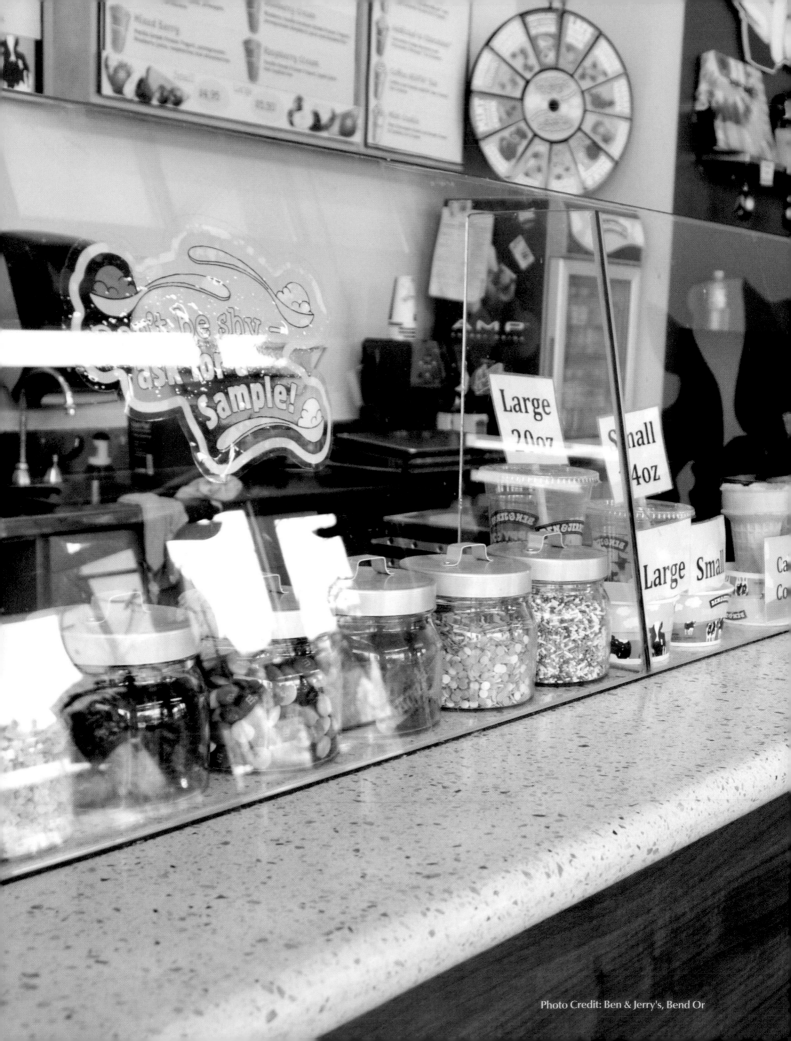

The Ice Cream Shop

Blood Orange Sorbet

Makes about 1 pint
Dairy Free • Egg Free • Fish Free • Nut Free

2 cups (475 mL) blood orange juice (about 6 large)

2 tsp blood orange zest

2 TBSP raw honey

2 TBSP coconut nectar

Squeeze fresh lime juice

Blood oranges sound and look a little on the "dark" side, but the flavor is out of this world! Very similar to a regular orange, but with an extra punch of flavor, they make for excellent sauces and desserts. This recipe is my favorite way to use blood oranges.

1. Place all ingredients in a small bowl and whisk to combine.

2. Chill in the fridge for at least 1 hour.

3. Pour mixture into a prepared ice cream maker and follow manufacturer's instructions.

4. Serve and enjoy!

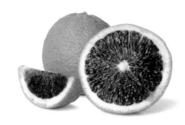

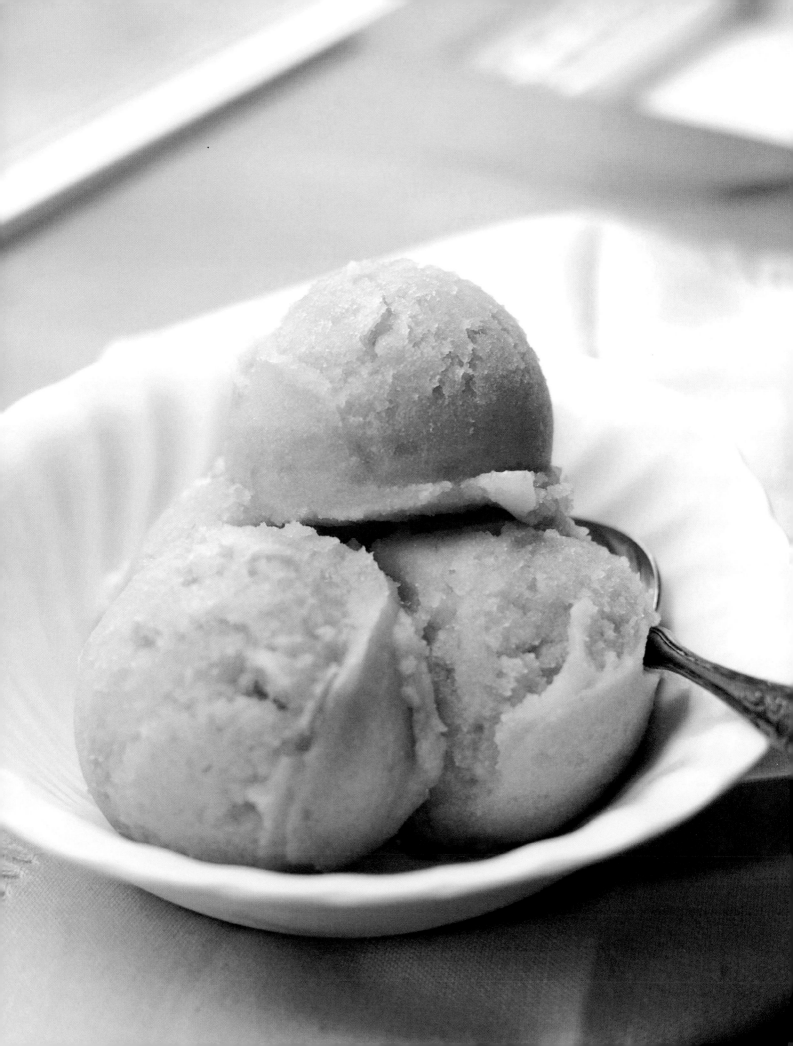

Coconut Colada Ice Cream

Makes about 1 pint
Dairy Free • Egg Free • Fish Free • Nut Free

Ice Cream

1 14-oz (400 mL) can coconut milk (full-fat or light)

2 small, ripe bananas (or 1 large)

1 cup (150 g) diced pineapple

Juice of 2 limes

¼-½ cup (22-45 g) unsweetened shredded coconut (vary depending on your taste)

Topping

½ cup (45 g) toasted unsweetened coconut flakes

This delicious tropical treat will make you feel like you are beach-side with every bite! You'll notice that there are no added sweeteners in this one—the fruit adds plenty of sweetness all by its lonesome. Make a batch on a nice, hot summer day and save a little to make popsicles. Then you can serve them to your kids with breakfast some morning and they'll think you've gone a little loco by giving them ice cream for break-fast! But you'll know you're really giving them something full of healthy ingredients, including good-quality fat from the coconut milk.

1. Place all the ice cream ingredients in a blender and purée until almost smooth. Slightly lumpy is good. Place in the refrigerator to cool, about 1 hour.

2. Pour mixture into a prepared ice cream maker and follow manufacturer's instructions for your machine.

3. Scoop into serving dishes and top with toasted coconut.

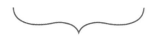

Note:
Toast the coconut by spreading it out in a thin layer on a baking sheet and baking in a 300°F oven 10-15 minutes, stirring every few minutes to help it toast evenly.

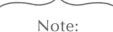

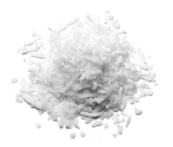

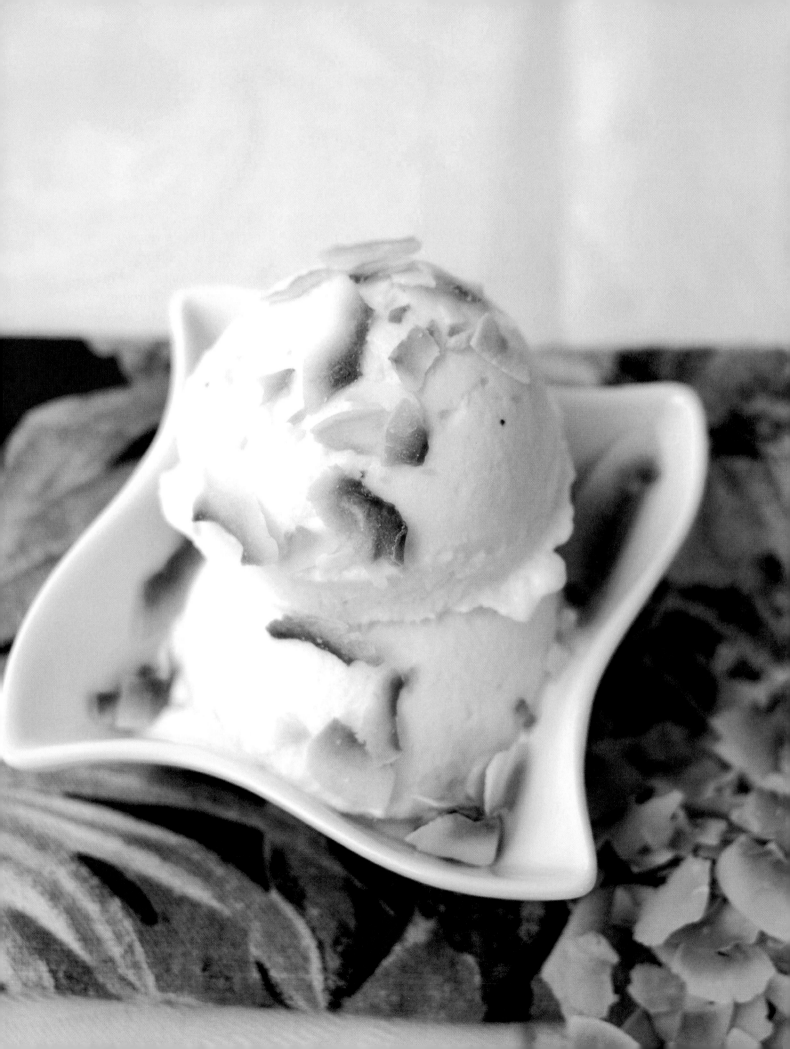

Kiwi Sorbet

Makes about 1 pint

Dairy Free • Egg Free • Fish Free • Nut Free

10 ripe kiwis, peeled

2 TBSP raw honey

2 TBSP coconut nectar

Squeeze fresh lime juice

I tried kiwi sorbet for the first time while visiting Disneyland last year. It topped off one of the best gluten-free Paleo meals we'd ever had at a restaurant, but I'm pretty sure it was loaded with sugar, as most treats in the non-Paleo world are. I wanted that same fresh flavor without the sugar-load and was very happy with my bright green results. Perfect for a summer afternoon. Or a Tuesday. Or now. Whatever works.

1. Place all ingredients in a blender or food processor and purée until smooth.

2. Chill in the fridge for at least 1 hour.

3. Pour the mixture into a prepared ice cream maker and follow manufacturer's instructions.

4. Serve and enjoy!

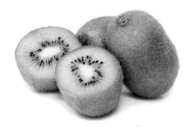

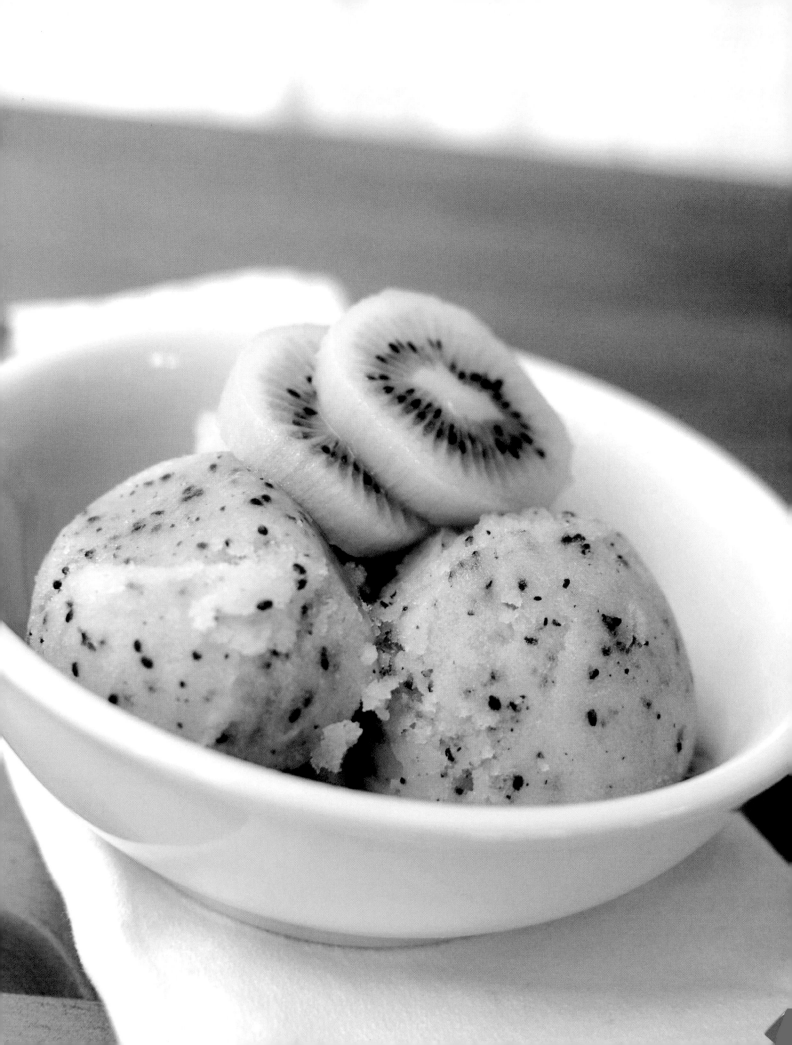

Mint-Chip Ice Cream

Makes about 1 pint
Dairy Free • Egg Free • Fish Free • Nut Free

1 14-oz (400 mL) can coconut milk (full-fat or light)

1 tsp pure vanilla extract

½ tsp pure peppermint extract

½ cup (75 g) raw spinach

⅓ cup (80 mL) pure maple syrup (or raw honey or coconut nectar)

½-¾ cup (80-120 g) dark chocolate shavings (depending on how chocolaty you want it)

We've made this minty treat for a couple of years now, but always left it white. Last Saint Patrick's Day, I wanted something fun for the kids after dinner, so I whipped up our typical ice cream but added spinach for color. Sure enough, the kiddos were thrilled with their bright green ice cream, and none the wiser that they also devoured a bunch of spinach! I think all parents have a right to be a little sneaky now and again. Keeps things interesting.

1. Place all ingredients, except the chocolate shavings, in a blender or food processor and purée until smooth.

2. Chill in the fridge for at least 1 hour.

3. Pour mixture into a prepared ice cream maker and follow manufacturer's instructions.

4. During the last 5 minutes of processing, add the chocolate shavings to the mixture.

5. Serve and enjoy!

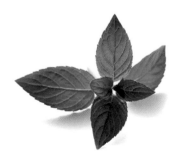

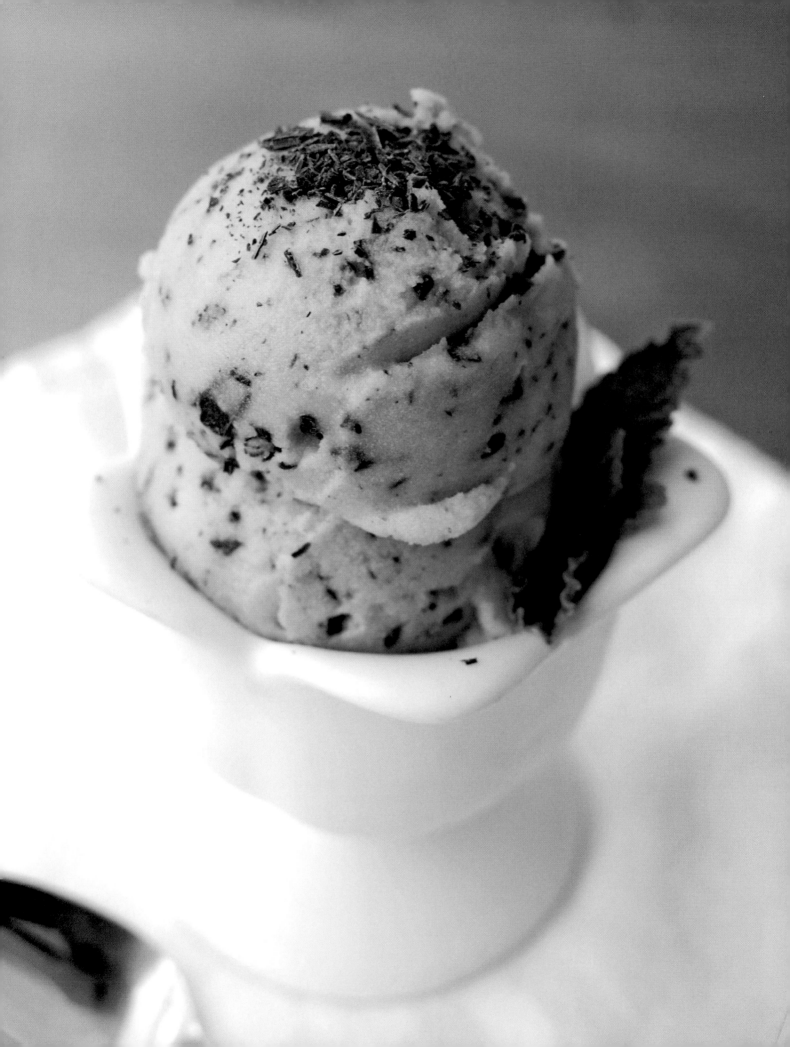

Orange Creamsicle

Makes about 1 pint

Dairy Free • Egg Free • Fish Free • Nut Free

1 14-oz (400 mL) can coconut milk (full-fat or light)

2 tsp pure vanilla extract

1 vanilla bean, split and scraped

½ cup (120 mL) orange juice concentrate

1 tsp orange zest

2 TBSP coconut nectar (or raw honey)

The perfect combination of orange and cream come together in this Paleo version of a 50/50 bar. Creamy yet light and refreshing, these'll keep you screaming for ice cream all summer!

1. Place all ingredients in a medium bowl and mix to combine. Refrigerate until cool, about 1 hour.

2. Pour the mixture into a prepared ice cream maker and follow manufacturer's instructions for your machine.

3. Scoop into serving dishes and enjoy!

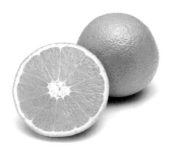

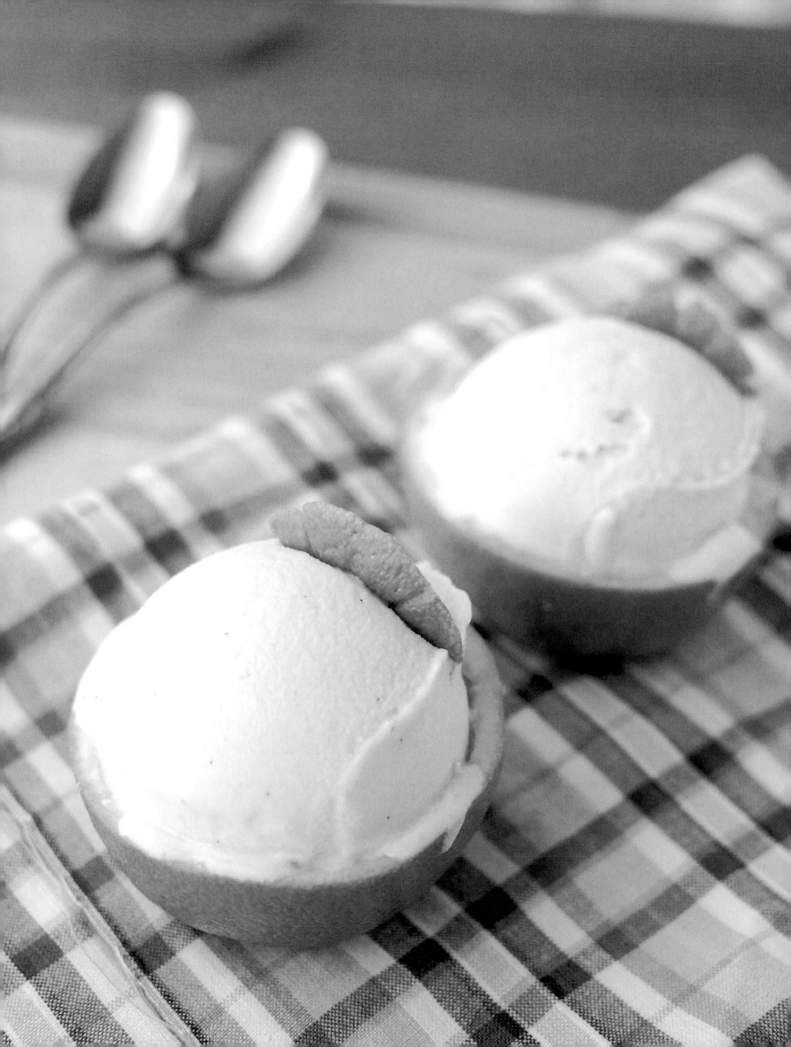

Pumpkin Pie-Sicle

Makes about 1 pint
Dairy Free • Egg Free • Fish Free • Nut Free

1 14-oz (400 mL) can coconut milk (full-fat or light)

²/₃ cup (160 g) canned pumpkin

2 tsp pure vanilla extract

¹/₃-¹/₂ cup (80-120 mL) pure maple syrup (depending on how sweet you want it)

1 tsp cinnamon

¼ tsp ginger

⅛ tsp nutmeg

Trick or treat! This creamy ice cream says fall is in the air, which means the holidays are just around the corner. So why not serve ice cream at Thanksgiving? It's like pumpkin pie in a bowl! This one is also delicious with a few dark chocolate chips added at the end.

1. Place all ingredients in a medium bowl and mix to combine. Refrigerate until cool, about 1 hour.

2. Pour the mixture into a prepared ice cream maker and follow manufacturer's instructions for your machine.

3. Scoop into serving dishes and enjoy!

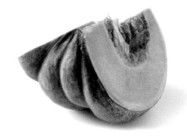

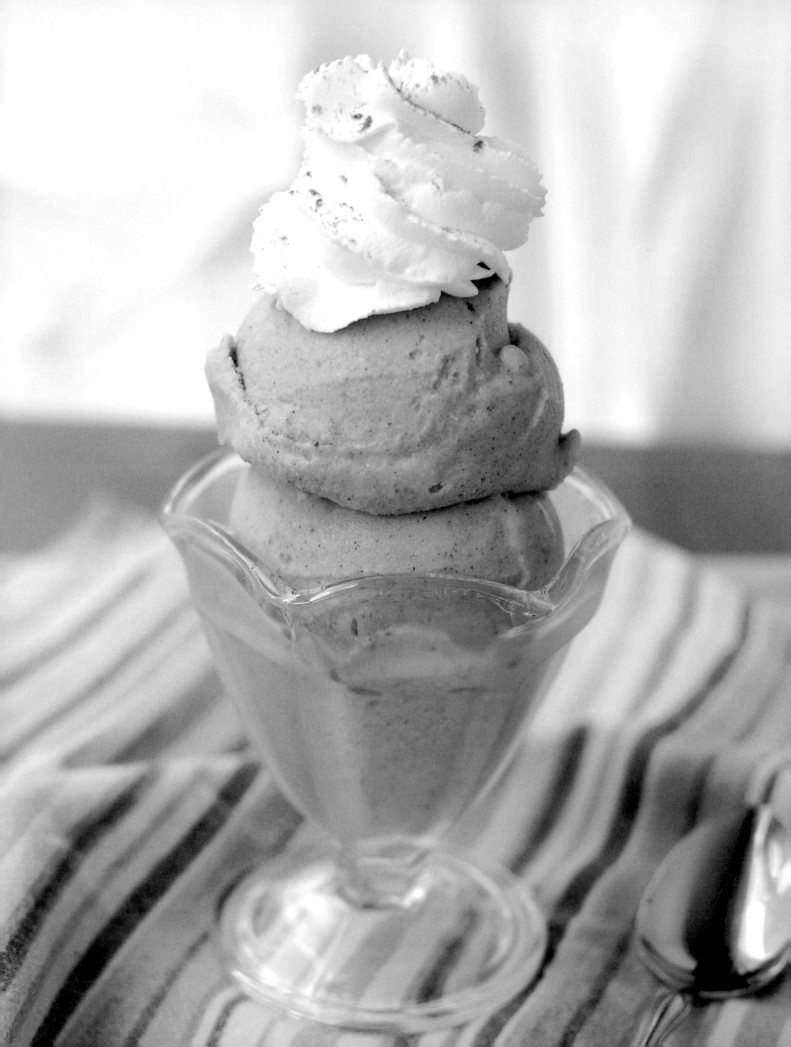

Like Magic Chocolate Ice Cream Topping

Makes about ¾ cup

Dairy Free • Egg Free • Fish Free • Nut Free

½ cup (120 mL) coconut oil, melted

2 TBSP unsweetened cocoa powder

¼ tsp pure vanilla extract

2 TBSP pure maple syrup

Pinch sea salt

Remember Magic Shell ice cream topping? Oh how I loooooved that chocolaty, crunchy coating! But as a kid, I was clueless about all the terrible ingredients. Eventually I wised up and did without for many years, until, that is, I concocted this, only slightly, sinful alternative! So here's the ice cream topping with all the crunch, chocolate, and great flavor I lived for as a kid without the trans-fats and corn syrup—that's what I call magic!

1. Place all ingredients in a medium bowl and whisk until cocoa powder is fully incorporated.

2. Spoon immediately over ice cream and watch it harden right before your eyes!

3. Store leftover topping in an airtight container in the fridge. To use, warm in the microwave until liquid, stir, and spoon over ice cream.

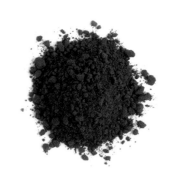

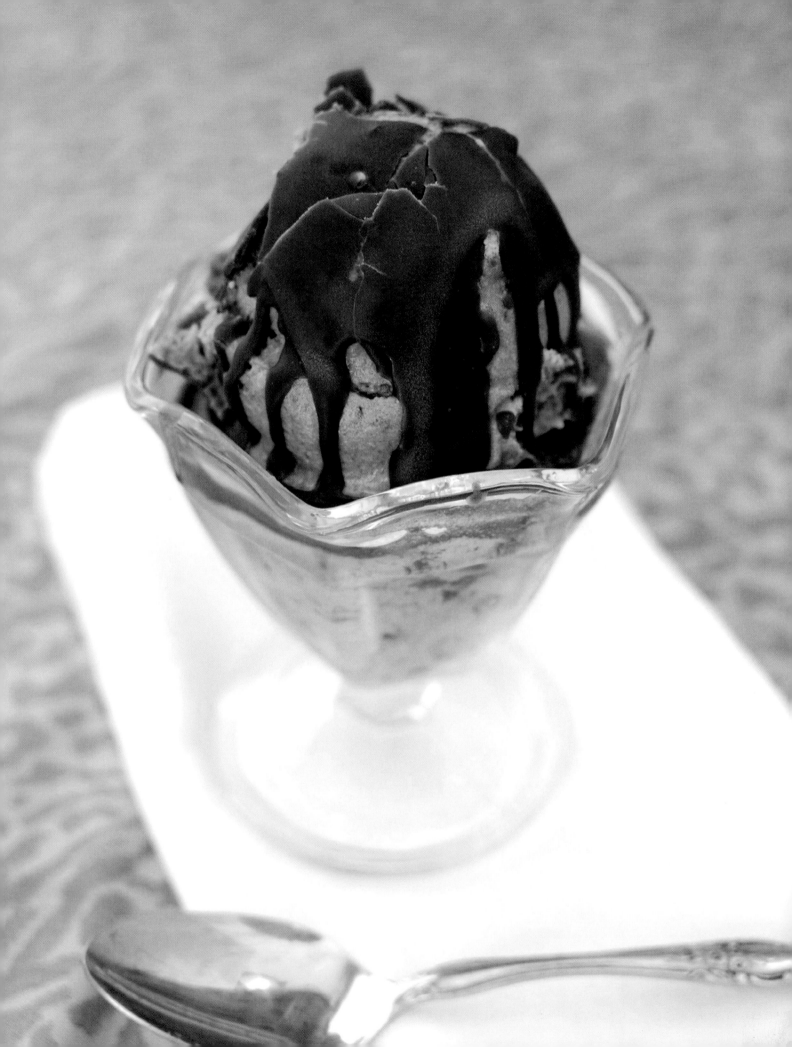

Shopping Resources

Azure Standard	http://www.azurestandard.com	Flavor extracts, honey, yeast, maple syrup, sea salt, cocoa powder, canned pumpkin, coconut oil, baking powder, baking soda, Spectrum organic palm shortening
Bob's Red Mill	http://www.bobsredmill.com	Arrowroot starch, coconut flour, almond meal, hazelnut meal
Coconut Secret	http://www.coconutsecret.com	Coconut aminos, coconut nectar, coconut crystals, coconut flour
Enjoy Life	http://www.enjoylifefoods.com	Mini chocolate chips and chocolate chunks (soy-free, dairy-free)
Flavorganics	http://www.flavorganics.com	Organic, non-GMO, gluten-free, all-natural extracts (vanilla, almond, peppermint, etc.)
Honeyville Farms	http://www.store.honeyvillegrain.com/blanchedalmondflour5lb.aspx	Blanched almond flour (certified gluten-free)
Let's Do Organic	http://www.edwardandsons.com/ldo_shop_coconut.itml	Coconut flakes, shredded coconut, creamed coconut (a.k.a. coconut butter)
Lodge Cast Iron	http://www.lodgemfg.com	Cast-iron cookware
McCormick	http://www.mccormick.com	Spices, but not spice blends, as McCormick doesn't guarantee that its blends are gluten-free, but its individual spices are
Really Raw Honey	http://www.reallyrawhoney.com	Raw, unprocessed honey
Thai Kitchen	http://www.thaikitchen.com/products/sauces-and-pastes/premium-fish-sauce.aspx	Premium fish sauce (gluten-free and dairy-free)
Trader Joe's	http://www.traderjoes.com, to find a store near you	Canned coconut milk; 72% organic, fair-trade dark chocolate; olive oil; nuts; seeds; organic fruits and veggies; unsweetened, unsulfured, dehydrated and freeze-dried fruits
Tropical Traditions	http://www.tropicaltraditions.com	Coconut oil and other coconut products
US Wellness Meat	http://www.grasslandbeef.com	Grass-fed, pastured meats
Whole Foods	http://www.wholefoodsmarket.com, to find a store near you	Red wine vinegar, balsamic vinegar, poppy seeds, sesame seeds, Spectrum organic palm shortening, olive oil, coconut oil, maple syrup, Dagoba unsweetened 100% chocolate, Enjoy Life chocolate chips, Bob's Red Mill flours, Coconut secret (aminos, nectar crystals, flour), coconut milk, Let's Do Organic (coconut flakes, shredded coconut, creamed coconut (aka coconut butter), sunbutter, almond butter, Fish sauce
Wilderness Family Naturals	http://www.wildernessfamilynaturals.com	Coconut oil and other coconut products
Wright's Natural Hickory Seasoning Liquid Smoke	http://www.bgfoods.com/wrights/	Natural, gluten-free, hickory-smoke flavoring

Farm & Information Resources

Eat Wild	http://www.eatwild.com	Information about, and links to, pastured, grass-fed meat products.
Weston A. Price Foundation	http://www.westonaprice.org	Information about the health benefits of organic, biodynamic farming and pasture-fed livestock.
The Healthy Gluten-Free Life	http://www.thehealthyglutenfreelife.com	From gluten-free to Paleo and all points in between. Find recipes, information and a dash of real-life experiences to help you on your journey to a healthier gluten-free life.
Eat Well Guide	http://www.eatwellguide.org	Where to find local, sustainable, organic food near you.
Local Harvest	http://www.localharvest.org	Where to find farmers' markets, family farms, CSAs (community supported agriculture), and other sources of sustainably grown food near you.

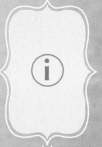

Ingredient Index

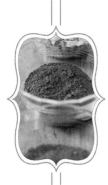

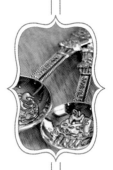

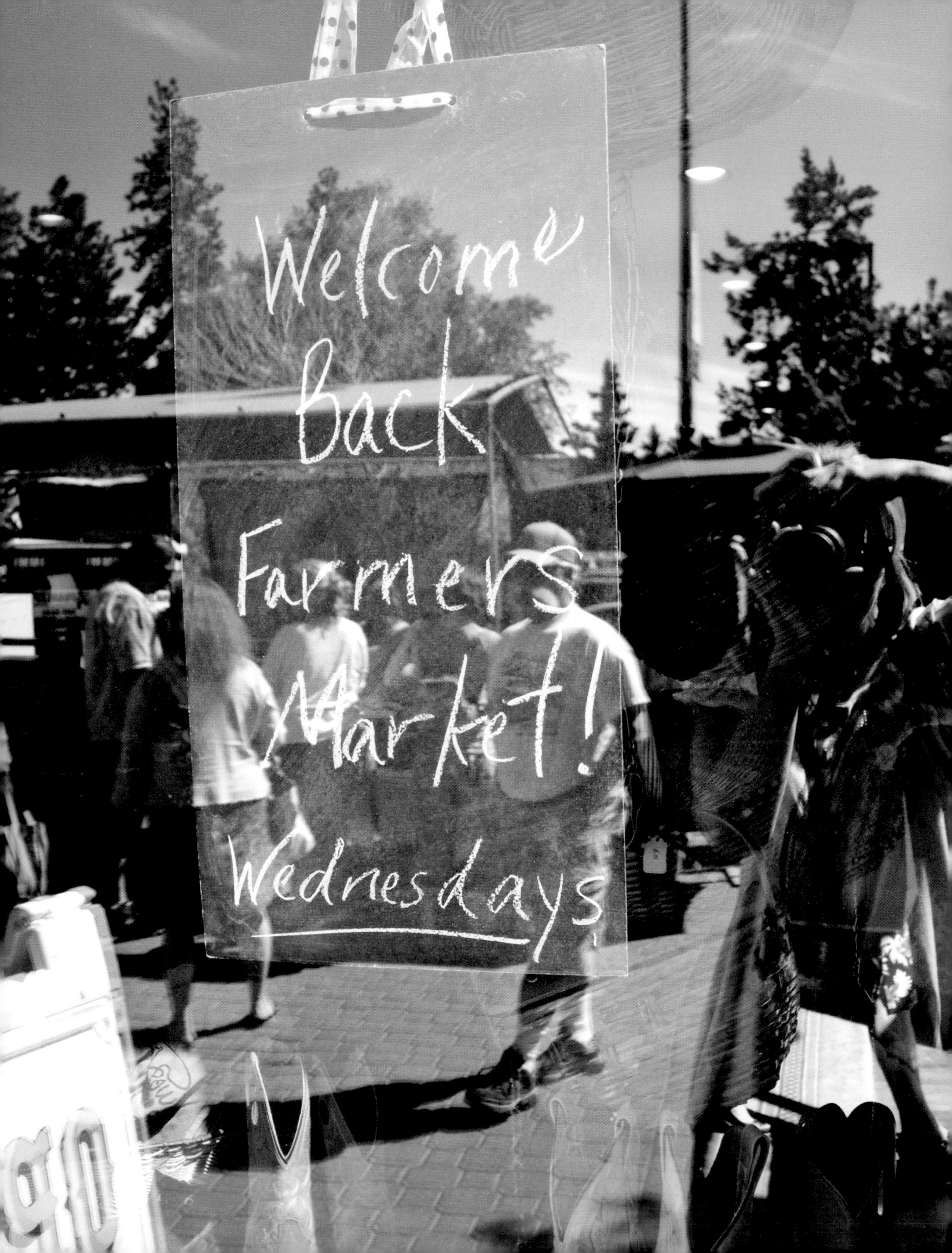
Welcome
Back
Farmers
Market!
Wednesdays

About the Author

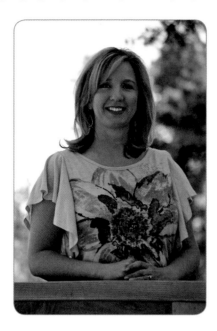

Tammy Credicott is a recipe developer and blogger and the author of *The Healthy Gluten-Free Life*. She and her husband owned a successful gluten-free, dairy-free, and egg-free bakery in Bend, Oregon, *The Celiac Maniac,* before they were inspired to transform their health further by switching to a Paleo lifestyle. Tammy has a passion for understanding health and wellness as it relates to nutrition and has used this knowledge to help her family overcome health issues such as celiac disease, food allergies, and ADD.

A self-taught home cook extraordinaire and Food Network junkie, she has transformed her family's well-being with the creation of simple, healthy, allergy-friendly—and delicious!—recipes that fit their busy lifestyle. And while some of her favorite things include summer vacation, months ending in "-ber," and photography, she finds her passion and enthusiasm for life in the kitchen with her family. Tammy lives in Bend, Oregon, with her husband and two daughters, and in her spare time, she likes to help her husband, Cain, with recipes and photography for *Paleo Magazine*, the only print magazine dedicated to the Paleo lifestyle and ancestral health.

http://www.facebook.com/thehealthygflife   https://twitter.com/healthygflife

https://www.thehealthyglutenfreelife.com

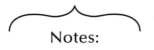

Notes:

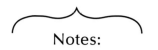
Notes:

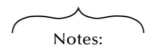

Notes:

Notes:

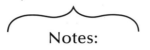
Notes: